# VACCINATING
## YOUR
## CHILD

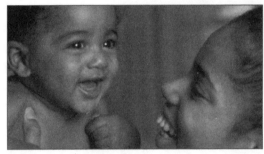

QUESTIONS &
ANSWERS FOR

## the concerned parent

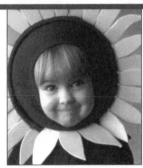

## Authors' Note

This book has been written as a resource for parents. Any information obtained here is not to be construed as medical or legal advice. Decisions about vaccination should be made on an individual basis after careful research and consultation with healthcare professionals who have expertise in childhood immunization.

Information in this book is based on the best data available as of Spring 2000. Talk to your healthcare professional because more information may be available now, and recommendations and scheduling may have changed.

Sharon G. Humiston
Cynthia Good

# VACCINATING
## YOUR
## CHILD

QUESTIONS &
ANSWERS FOR
## the concerned parent

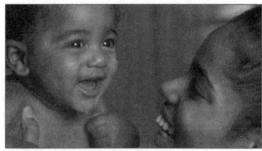

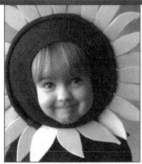

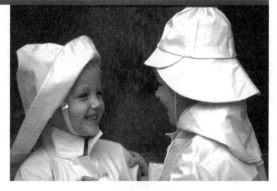

**Sharon G. Humiston**, M.D., M.P.H.

**Cynthia Good**

PEACHTREE
ATLANTA

A happy family is but an earlier heaven.

I dedicate this book to my husband Joey and my boys Alden and Julien
who give me a shot of love, support, and salvation every single day.
They are my everything.

—C. G.

Glad for Spring, we,
as one, slide melting panes aside
to let the swallow sail.

—S. G. H.

Published by
PEACHTREE PUBLISHERS, LTD.
1700 Chattahoochee Avenue
Atlanta, Georgia 30318-2112

*www.peachtree-online.com*

Text © 2000 by Sharon G. Humiston and Cynthia Good
Cover photographs © 2000, Bill Tucker Studio, Inc.: child doctor, raincoat kids, flower child; James
Davis: nurse and baby. Photos via International Stock, New York, NY.

This book was written by Sharon G. Humiston in her private capacity. No official support or endorsement by CDC is intended or should be inferred. All interviews were conducted by Cynthia Good.

Book and cover design by Loraine M. Balcsik
Book composition by Melanie M. McMahon

Manufactured in the United States of America

10 9 8 7 6 5 4

Library of Congress Cataloging-in-Publication Data

Humiston, Sharon
    Vaccinating your child : questions and answers for the concerned parent /
    Sharon Humiston and Cynthia Good.
        p. cm.
    ISBN 1-56145-177-0
        1. Vaccination of children--Miscellanea. 2. Communicable diseases--
    Prevention--Miscellanea. I. Good, Cynthia. II. Title.

RA638 .H36 2000
614.4'7'083--dc21                                          99-462007

# Contents

# PART THREE  What You Should Know about Other Vaccines

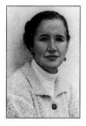

Dr. Sharon G. Humiston received her M.D. from the Medical College of Ohio and her M.P.H. from the University of Rochester. She is a Medical Epidemiologist in the Training and Education Branch of the Immunization Services Division of the National Immunization Program at the Centers for Disease Control and Prevention. Dr. Humiston brings to this project a wealth of information, having served as a board-certified pediatrician doing immunization research with the CDC since 1989. She is also a member of the clinical faculty at the University of Rochester Medical Center.

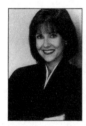

Cynthia Good, an award-winning journalist and television news reporter, attended Sarah Lawrence College and received her B.A. in Political Science at UCLA. Ms. Good's experiences as a journalist and more recently as the creator and host of the television show *Good for Parents* were valuable resources in the researching and writing of this book. She is also the author of the best selling book *Words Every Child Must Hear*.

For several years Ms. Good and Dr. Humiston have participated together in live videoconferences from the CDC to public healthcare providers across the U.S., Mexico, and Canada. This series of broadcasts has focused on the latest developments in childhood vaccines.

As mothers of young children, both authors have a personal as well as a professional interest in the topic of immunizations.

# Acknowledgments

We would like to offer our special thanks to the parents and colleagues whom we have spoken with, and without whose help this publication would not have been possible.

Many thanks go to the people who graciously shared their knowledge, experience, and insight, including those from CDC National Immunization Program, William Atkinson, Kris Bisgard, Beth Hibbs, Dean Mason, Gina Mootrey, Walter Orenstein, Lance Rodewald, Chuck Vitek, Bruce Weniger, and Skip Wolfe; from CDC National Center for Infectious Diseases, Eric Mast; from the Center for Biologics Evaluation & Research, FDA, Peter A. Patriarca.

To the public health experts from many states: Gillian Stoltman and Nancy Fasano in Michigan; Trang Kuss and Cynthia Gleason in Washington; Deborah Jelks in Georgia; Bob Crider and Jan Pelosi in Texas; Doug Lyon in Utah. To Muriel Colstock, fourth year pharmacy student. To those from the Immunization Action Coalition, Deborah Wexler; and from Medimmune, Rip Ballou. And to the many parents who shared their stories.

Margaret Quinlin, our publisher, richly deserves our thanks as the first who believed in us and in our idea. Thanks also go to our editor, Sarah Helyar Smith, who smilingly helped turn what we wrote into English; and to Vicky Holifield, copy editor, Melanie McMahon, associate production manager, and Loraine Balcsik, art director, who all waded through many drafts to make sure that this book turned out well.

We send our thanks to our family and friends for their constant encouragement. From Cynthia, a heartfelt thanks to Joey, Alden, and Julien Reiman and friends Sara and Armand Harris, Denise and Mark Connolly, Meg Reggie, Arthur and Lois Cohen, and Craig and Amy Weil. Also, thanks to Glen and Elaine Good, and Bob and Kathy Good. From Sharon, thanks to Mom and Dad for teaching me my first words; to Nancy and Bruce, Doris and Donald for cheering words; to Sue and Nancy for their intimacies dressed in words, and to Bob, Jocelyn, and Quinn for their wordless communication. Our gratitude also goes to Barbara Briggs for her therapeutic gifts—both insightful and aromatic in nature.

Ultimately, our thanks flow to the Source of all life and all support.

# PART ONE

## Vaccine Use

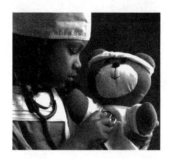

*My experience in government is that when things are non-controversial
and beautifully coordinated, there is not much going on.*

—John Fitzgerald Kennedy

*Knowledge is power.*

—Francis Bacon

Chapter 1

# Introduction

This is an historic time for childhood vaccines. Nowadays, a parent is more likely to know someone who had a vaccine side effect than someone who had one of the old vaccine-preventable diseases (such as tetanus or diphtheria). Because of the success of vaccines, American parents and healthcare providers have less experience than ever before with infectious diseases such as polio and measles. At the same time, more vaccines are universally recommended, and new vaccines are being introduced for diseases that many people had previously considered a normal part of life, like diarrhea and chickenpox. News stories about vaccine safety appear one after another. Consider the summer of 1999, when all of these stories hit the press:

- ✛ The CDC and the American Academy of Pediatrics, which had previously recommended rotavirus vaccine to prevent diarrhea in infants, postponed further use of the vaccine when data showed that the vaccine was causing bowel obstruction.

- ✛ After questions were raised about the safety of thimerosal (a mercury-containing preservative used in many vaccines), pharmaceutical companies began complying quickly with governmental and medical calls to eliminate the mercury, but the preservative-free vaccines cost significantly more.

✥ With the long-anticipated global eradication of polio close at hand, the U.S. returned to primary reliance on the injectable polio vaccine. Why? Because the vaccine given by mouth, which has been used since the mid-1960s, caused 8 to 10 cases of paralytic disease each year.

✥ Congressional hearings were held because of allegations that hepatitis B vaccine was too unsafe to be included in the routine childhood immunization schedule.

✥ The Department of Defense ordered active military forces and reservists to accept the anthrax vaccine because of bioterrorist threats, but some individuals chose court martial over compliance because they feared complications from the vaccine.

These factors have combined to fuel a growing sense of confusion, concern, and frustration among parents. Will these controversies increase the proportion of American children who do not receive vaccines? Will states relax their school entry laws? Will infectious diseases return to devastate our children? Will we realize that our fears were unfounded? When the same immunizations that have saved so many lives are being blamed for everything from autism to multiple sclerosis, from asthma to sudden infant death syndrome, parents aren't sure where to turn for answers, or even what questions to ask.

## TO VACCINATE OR NOT TO VACCINATE?

That is not the question! All too often parents ask, "Are you for or against vaccination?" as if all vaccines were created equally and as if all infectious diseases were similar. As you read the chapters about individual diseases, you will see some similarities, but you will learn about the important details that distinguish the diseases from each other and the particulars that differentiate the vaccines.

And you will see that the information provided is *useful*. For example, after reading this book you may feel it is important to do the following:

- ✛ Know if your child has a medical reason not to receive a vaccine.

- ✛ Know the most common side effects of the vaccines your child is given and be prepared to treat them.

- ✛ Be aware of and alert to rare vaccine side effects.

- ✛ If you are pregnant, be sure that your obstetrician checks your blood for hepatitis B infection at the end of pregnancy and, if the test is positive, that your newborn receives hepatitis B vaccine and hepatitis B immune globulin within twelve hours after birth.

- ✛ Be sure that the medical practice your child goes to uses the newer, "acellular" pertussis vaccine.

- ✛ Be sure that your child is given only the injectable polio vaccine.

- ✛ Be sure that the physician checks your teenager's blood for chickenpox immunity and, if the test is negative, gives the chickenpox vaccine.

## NOT THE LAST WORD

This book contains the most recent data available, as of Spring 2000, on each of the vaccines and on vaccine-preventable diseases, but no book could contain all the information you need. We do not intend this to be the last word on immunization. Rather, our intention is simply to prepare you for initiating a conversation about immunization with your child's healthcare provider. Ultimately, we believe there is no good substitute for a trustworthy healthcare provider with whom you can openly discuss your vaccine questions.

Although most parents feel comfortable with their children's physicians, they are reluctant to ask questions or enter into a discussion. This is unfortunate because children receive the best healthcare when parents and physicians work in partnership. To be in a partnership, *you* have to be a partner.

## PERMISSION GRANTED

Studies on doctor-patient communication done by a prominent health education research team at Louisiana State University confirmed what might seem like common sense to a parent. The team found that parents wanted information on vaccine risks and benefits and that they would not reflexively reject vaccines after these factors were explained. In focus groups, parents expressed the desire to have materials to read in advance of office visits because the visit itself was too hectic a time to *start* thinking about vaccine issues.

The research team created a colorful poster that suggested some questions parents should ask and hung the poster in pediatric exam rooms. Preliminary studies showed that the poster did make a difference: parents were more likely to ask questions about vaccine safety after reading the poster and were more satisfied with the visit. Further research on the effectiveness of this approach is being pursued.

Of course, what the poster *really* did was to remind parents of their questions and, probably more importantly, to give parents permission or encouragement to ask their vaccine questions.

## YOUR RIGHT TO KNOW

Actually, in 1986 the federal government gave all parents—poster or not—the *right* to know what benefits and risks their children face with each vaccine. Your healthcare provider is required by federal law to provide you with this information, even if you don't ask for it. According to the National Childhood Vaccine Injury Act of 1986, your healthcare provider also is required to give you Vaccine Information Statements, one-page summaries of specific vaccine risks and benefits published by the CDC. (See Figure 1-1 for a sample of the MMR vaccine handout.) Receipt of the written summary and discussion of it must precede every routine childhood vaccination because the information is frequently updated. If you are not given this information, ask for it! Asking for the information is your responsibility; getting it is your right.

# MEASLES MUMPS & RUBELLA VACCINES

## W H A T   Y O U   N E E D   T O   K N O W

### 1  Why get vaccinated?

Measles, mumps, and rubella are serious diseases.

**Measles**
- Measles virus causes rash, cough, runny nose, eye irritation, and fever.
- It can lead to ear infection, pneumonia, seizures (jerking and staring), brain damage, and death.

**Mumps**
- Mumps virus causes fever, headache, and swollen glands.
- It can lead to deafness, meningitis (infection of the brain and spinal cord covering), painful swelling of the testicles or ovaries, and, rarely, death.

**Rubella (German Measles)**
- Rubella virus causes rash, mild fever, and arthritis (mostly in women).
- If a woman gets rubella while she is pregnant, she could have a miscarriage or her baby could be born with serious birth defects.

You or your child could catch these diseases by being around someone who has them. They spread from person to person through the air.

**Measles, mumps, and rubella (MMR) vaccine can prevent these diseases.**

Most children who get their MMR shots will not get these diseases. Many more children would get them if we stopped vaccinating.

### 2  Who should get MMR vaccine and when?

Children should get 2 doses of MMR vaccine:

✓ The first at 12-15 months of age
✓ and the second at 4-6 years of age.

These are the recommended ages. But children can get the second dose at any age, as long as it is at least 28 days after the first dose.

Some adults should also get MMR vaccine:

Generally, anyone 18 years of age or older, who was born after 1956, should get at least one dose of MMR vaccine, unless they can show that they have had either the vaccines or the diseases.

Ask your doctor or nurse for more information.

MMR vaccine may be given at the same time as other vaccines.

### 3  Some people should not get MMR vaccine or should wait

- People should not get MMR vaccine who have ever had a life-threatening allergic reaction to **gelatin**, the antibiotic **neomycin**, or a **previous dose of MMR vaccine.**

- People who are moderately or severely ill at the time the shot is scheduled usually should wait until they recover before getting MMR vaccine.

- Pregnant women should wait to get MMR vaccine until after they have given birth. Women should not get pregnant for 3 months after getting MMR vaccine.

- Some people should check with their doctor about whether they should get MMR vaccine, including anyone who:
  - Has HIV/AIDS, or another disease that affects the immune system
  - Is being treated with drugs that affect the immune system, such as steroids, for 2 weeks or longer.
  - Has any kind of cancer
  - Is taking cancer treatment with x-rays or drugs
  - Has ever had a low platelet count (a blood disorder)

*Over . . .*

- People who recently had a transfusion or were given other blood products should ask their doctor when they may get MMR vaccine

Ask your doctor or nurse for more information.

### 4  What are the risks from MMR vaccine?

A vaccine, like any medicine, is capable of causing serious problems, such as severe allergic reactions. The risk of MMR vaccine causing serious harm, or death, is extremely small.

Getting MMR vaccine is much safer than getting any of these three diseases.

Most people who get MMR vaccine do not have any problems with it.

**Mild Problems**
- Fever (up to 1 person out of 6)
- Mild rash (about 1 person out of 20)
- Swelling of glands in the cheeks or neck (rare)
If these problems occur, it is usually within 7-12 days after the shot. They occur less often after the second dose.

**Moderate Problems**
- Seizure (jerking or staring) caused by fever (about 1 out of 3,000 doses)
- Temporary pain and stiffness in the joints, mostly in teenage or adult women (up to 1 out of 4)
- Temporary low platelet count, which can cause a bleeding disorder (about 1 out of 30,000 doses)

**Severe Problems (Very Rare)**
- Serious allergic reaction (less than 1 out of a million doses)
- Several other severe problems have been known to occur after a child gets MMR vaccine. But this happens so rarely, experts cannot be sure whether they are caused by the vaccine or not. These include:
  - Deafness
  - Long-term seizures, coma, or lowered consciousness
  - Permanent brain damage

### 5  What if there is a moderate or severe reaction?

**What should I look for?**

Any unusual conditions, such as a serious allergic reaction, high fever or behavior changes. Signs of a serious allergic reaction include difficulty breathing, hoarseness or wheezing, hives, paleness, weakness, a fast heart beat or dizziness within a few minutes to a few hours after the shot. A high fever or seizure, if it occurs, would happen 1 or 2 weeks after the shot.

**What should I do?**
- Call a doctor, or get the person to a doctor right away.
- Tell your doctor what happened, the date and time it happened, and when the vaccination was given.
- Ask your doctor, nurse, or health department to file a Vaccine Adverse Event Reporting System (VAERS) form, or call VAERS yourself at **1-800-822-7967.**

### 6  The National Vaccine Injury Compensation Program

In the rare event that you or your child has a serious reaction to a vaccine, a federal program has been created to help you pay for the care of those who have been harmed.

For details about the National Vaccine Injury Compensation Program, call **1-800-338-2382** or visit the program's website at **http://www.hrsa.dhhs.gov/bhpr/vicp**

### 7  How can I learn more?

- Ask your doctor or nurse. They can give you the vaccine package insert or suggest other sources of information.
- Call your local or state health department's immunization program.
- Contact the Centers for Disease Control and Prevention (CDC):
  - Call **1-800-232-2522** (English)
  - Call **1-800-232-0233** (Español)
  - Visit the National Immunization Program's website at **http://www.cdc.gov/nip**

**U.S. DEPARTMENT OF HEALTH & HUMAN SERVICES**
Centers for Disease Control and Prevention
National Immunization Program

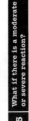

Vaccine Information Statement

MMR (12/16/98)          42 U.S.C. § 300aa-26

**Figure 1-1**
## SAMPLE VACCINE HANDOUT: MMR

## THE GOALS OF THIS BOOK

Our goals are twofold. *First,* we want to empower you to ask your healthcare provider questions about vaccines. In fact, everyone from every corner of the vaccine debate wants you to ask questions. Chances are quite high that your healthcare provider also wants you to ask.

*Second,* we want to give you the most recent scientific information on vaccine-preventable diseases and on the vaccines themselves. We hope you will use this book to prepare for your child's routine doctor visits. You'll soon know what shots your child is likely to receive, their possible side effects, and their benefits, so you can make your own informed decisions about vaccinating your child.

## USING THIS BOOK TO FORM AND ANSWER YOUR QUESTIONS

We have designed the book for busy parents (parents are busy by definition!), breaking it into three parts.

Part One gives you background on vaccines: what you should expect from your healthcare provider's immunization services; how vaccines work with your immune system; how vaccines are developed, licensed, recommended, and finally required for school entry; how programs track vaccine side effects over the long run; how to analyze vaccine risks; and who should *not* receive specific vaccines.

Part Two discusses the specific vaccines that your child will probably need to receive before attending school.

Part Three reviews vaccines that are not *routinely* recommended for children and vaccines that *are* recommended for adolescents and adults. Finally, because you may find that new questions come to mind, the last chapter lists some organizations that you might want to contact. We believe that the single most reliable and accessible source for quick answers is the CDC hotline: (800) 232-2522.

*The only way to keep your health is to eat what you don't want,*
*drink what you don't like, and do what you'd rather not.*

—Mark Twain

# Chapter 2

# Doctor Visits: What to Expect

Most parents would rather not see (or hear) their children being vaccinated, and children, who never before have faced so many vaccinations, certainly don't want to have the injections. By the time they enter school, children in the U.S. today receive more than 30 doses of vaccine in as many as 20 separate injections. When you visit your child's healthcare provider, you'll probably find that these vaccines are taken for granted as one of the key elements of well-child care, although they are neither 100 percent safe nor 100 percent effective. If vaccines are not perfectly safe and effective, why do we put our children through this? The answer has to do with the devastation caused by diseases most of us don't even remember.

The good old days were not so good in a lot of ways. Ask your grandmother what it was like to raise children when poliovirus was rampaging through the U.S., paralyzing more than 20,000 people in a single year (see Chapter 10). The fear of this invader was pervasive because, like AIDS today, polio caused long-term disabilities and death; but unlike AIDS, polio *was* spread through casual contact within homes and schools and public restrooms. If your physician is older than 40, ask him or her what it was like to care for children limp and lethargic with meningitis from Hib (see Chapter 11), knowing that, even if the antibiotics did work, the child still had a 15 to 30 percent risk of permanent nervous system damage. Before vaccines, grandmothers used to exhort new mothers, "Don't count your children until they have survived measles." Ask a nurse how parents *demanded* measles vaccine during the outbreak in the early 1990s when 123 U.S. children died from measles, right here in the wealthiest, most technologically advanced country in the world.

While most parents and healthcare providers agree that vaccination is worth doing, many parents and healthcare providers might be confused about how to do it well. What vaccines should be given? When? Where? What are the precautions?

## The Recommended Childhood Immunization Schedule

Most healthcare providers vaccinate their young patients according to a schedule similar to the one shown in Table 2-1 as recommended by the American Academy of Pediatrics (AAP), the American Academy of Family Physicians (AAFP), and the Advisory Committee on Immunization Practices (ACIP), an independent board that advises CDC.

The schedule shown reflects one commonly used pattern for vaccine timing, but there is flexibility in the scheduling of many vaccines. For example, the first dose of hepatitis B vaccine is recommended for use any time between birth and 2 months of age; the fourth dose of DTaP is recommended at 12 to 18 months of age.

States do not require vaccination until entry in daycare, Head Start, or school, so if you feel strongly about delaying protection against certain diseases, it is possible to do so. (See a detailed discussion on page 53.)

## Preparing for the Visit

### Keeping good vaccination records

Most of us are so busy that we have trouble remembering if we fed the kids lunch, let alone if we had them vaccinated two years ago. Keep an up-to-date immunization record for your child. Not only will that help ensure that your child does not miss any vaccinations, but it will also mean that

Table 2-1

## YEAR 2000 ROUTINE CHILDHOOD IMMUNIZATION SCHEDULE

| Child's Age | Routine Vaccines Given[1] | | | |
|---|---|---|---|---|
| Birth | hepatitis B | | | |
| 2 Months | | DTaP | Hib | polio shot | pneumococcal |
| 4 Months | hepatitis B | DTaP | Hib | polio shot | pneumococcal |
| 6 Months | hepatitis B | DTaP | (Hib)[2] | | pneumococcal |
| 12 Months | | | Hib | | MMR, chickenpox |
| 15 Months | | DTaP | | polio shot | pneumococcal |
| 24 Months | hepatitis A[3] | | | | |
| 4-6 Years | | DTaP | | polio shot | MMR |
| 11-12 Years and every 10 years thereafter | | Td | | | |

DTaP: Diphtheria, tetanus, and acellular pertussis vaccine

Td: Tetanus and diphtheria vaccine (for adolescents and adults)

Hib: *Haemophilus influenzae* type b vaccine

Polio shot: The "shot" is inactivated polio vaccine, IPV

MMR: Measles, mumps, and rubella vaccine

[1] The schedule shown reflects one commonly used pattern for vaccine timing, but there is flexibility in the scheduling of many vaccines. For example, the first dose of hepatitis B vaccine may be given at 2 months of age and the fourth dose of DTaP may be given at 12 to 18 months of age. Some vaccines may be given as combinations (e.g., DTaP-Hib at 12-15 months or Hepatitis B-Hib after 6 weeks of age).

[2] The 6-month dose of Hib is not needed with one brand of the vaccine.

[3] Hepatitis A vaccine is recommended for children living in certain states. Most experts recommend two doses. Please see the Hepatitis A chapter (14) and talk to your local healthcare provider.

*Source: ACIP*

you don't have to contact the doctor's office every time a school, camp, or club wants a copy. Keep in mind that if your child's medical record is lost, he or she may have to start all over with the vaccination series before being allowed to enroll in school. We have included immunization records inside the front and back covers of this book for your use.

Whatever immunization record card you use, keep it with you, and have the doctor's office update it after each visit. Or you can wait until your child has completed the preschool series at about 4 to 6 years of age, then get a photocopy of the completed immunization record from the doctor's office, make additional copies, and store them in something you will not lose—like your telephone book or wedding album, or this book.

### Reminders and recall messages

While we are reminded when to visit the dentist, the vet, or even the auto mechanic, we are rarely reminded of important doctor visits. At 2 years of age and thereafter, your child's birthday serves as an annual reminder, but you will need something to help you remember office visits the rest of the year. Encourage your child's health care provider to send a reminder. Additionally, if your child misses an appointment when vaccines were scheduled, make sure to reschedule the visit.

## FINDING OUT ABOUT THE VACCINE

### Getting your questions answered

Federal law requires healthcare providers to discuss the risks and benefits of each vaccine before it is given, so if your child's pediatrician doesn't take the initiative on this, make sure that you do. The doctor or nurse will be glad to provide details, but you are more likely to remember to ask questions if you have written them down beforehand. (You might want to read this book with a pen and pad handy.)

### Screening before vaccination

Not all children should receive all vaccines. For example, a child who has had a serious allergic reaction to DTaP vaccine should not receive it again. Ask your healthcare provider to screen your child before vaccination to see if there are any reasons to hold off on one or more vaccines. A simple screening checklist that you and your healthcare provider may find helpful appears in Chapter 6, where we discuss in detail why some children should not receive certain vaccines. In each vaccine chapter we list the reasons why a person might not be a good candidate for that vaccine.

## Before, During, and After the Shot

### Pain control: Needle tips

Numbing medications for the skin (such as EMLA Cream, which takes 45 minutes to work, or Vapocoolant Spray, which works on contact) have been shown to decrease the pain of the injection. Acetaminophen or ibuprofen, but *not* aspirin, can be given at the very beginning of the visit to lessen muscle aches after the injection, but these do little for the pain of the needle itself.

Some techniques that do not involve medicines have been shown to decrease injection pain. For example, firm pressure to the injection site before and after the shot can lessen the discomfort. Some children can simply be distracted from the pain. If your child has special difficulty tolerating injections, you may wish to consult a capable medical hypnotist.

### Where and how much vaccine should be given

MMR and chickenpox vaccines are injected just under the skin. The polio shot, IPV, may be given this way or, like all the other vaccines in the routine schedule, injected into muscles of the upper arm or thigh. DTaP, Hib, pneumococcal, and hepatitis B vaccines should be injected only into these muscles; if they are injected just under the skin there is more likelihood of pain, swelling, and redness at the site.

Stop anyone who is preparing your child's buttock for an injection! No one should receive a vaccination in the buttocks, because a large nerve that runs through the buttock muscles can be damaged by the needle. Also, a vaccine that is supposed to be injected into a muscle is much less likely to be effective if it ends up short of the mark—that is, if it is injected into the fat that lies on top of the muscles of the buttocks. Because vaccines given improperly may not work, the immunization advisory board to CDC recommends *repeating* a vaccine dose given in a nonstandard place (for instance, if your child received hepatitis B vaccine in the buttocks) or by a nonstandard route (for instance, if DTaP was given under the skin instead of into a muscle).

Some physicians have tried to reduce the number of side effects (especially when giving the old pertussis vaccines) by splitting doses. There was never any evidence that this practice actually reduced the number of side effects, and administering half a dose now and the other half on another day *may not work at all*.

## Handling side effects

Many children are uncomfortable after receiving vaccines. They're fussy and may have a fever or a red, swollen, tender area where the injection was given. Two over-the-counter medicines, acetaminophen (such as Tylenol™) and ibuprofen (such as Advil™), are commonly used to help children with these problems. Acetaminophen can be used every four hours and ibuprofen can be used every six hours.

Parents often ask if there is a danger of masking a fever that develops after the vaccine, but fever by itself is not worrisome, just uncomfortable. When doctors seem concerned about signs of illness accompanied by fever, they are concerned because the fever may be a signal that the immune system is gearing up against a real infection. Fever soon after some vaccines (such as DTaP or hepatitis B vaccine) is not uncommon and is only a signal that the immune system is gearing up against the vaccine, which is exactly what the doctor wants it to do.

A small bag of ice on a sore injection site may help with pain and keep the inflammation down. A cool, clean, wet cloth is also helpful. A bath with lukewarm, not cold, water may make a child with a fever more comfortable.

Of course, if your child suffers a serious side effect, such as a seizure, call your doctor or emergency medical service immediately. You should report side effects to your child's doctor and to the Vaccine Adverse Event Reporting System (see Chapter 4).

## CONCLUSION

The meek may inherit the earth, but they and their children may not get the best healthcare before then. If you are concerned about how your child is receiving vaccines at your doctor's office, then speak to the doctor about it. No matter how much knowledge and sensitivity your doctors and nurses display, no one is a better advocate for your child than you are.

*Every advance in civilization has been denounced as unnatural while it was recent.*

—Bertrand Russell

# Chapter 3

# How Vaccines Work with the Immune System

Some critics of vaccination chide that the "unnatural" practice of vaccination ignores or tricks our immune systems. Quite to the contrary, the success of vaccination relies completely upon having a healthy immune system. Vaccines work *with* the natural immune system, depending on the whole, intricate natural process. From the earliest inoculations—administered by a Chinese nun in the 1100s—to modern baby shots, vaccines only work as well as the immune system of the recipient.

## THE IMMUNE SYSTEM

Analogies are powerful. A good analogy is useful for illustrating a point. But sometimes people overextend or read too much into analogies, often ending up far from the truth. When talking about the immune system, a lot of people use words like "weak" or "strong." It is fine to use these descriptions that make the immune system sound like a muscle, but we should not take this analogy too far. A muscle atrophies if not used; the immune system does not. A muscle becomes exhausted by overuse; the immune system does not.

It is more useful, and more accurate, to compare the body's immune system to a loyal, intelligent, and powerful watchdog that ejects intruders from a home. The intruders, chiefly viruses and bacteria, enter the body through the nose, mouth, or broken skin. A healthy immune system recognizes the intruders as they begin to multiply in the lungs, bowels, or blood and destroys them.

A sound immune system distinguishes what belongs (healthy cells) from what doesn't (viruses and bacteria that invade the body from outside, or cancer cells that develop inside the body). A faulty immune system either allows invaders to wander unchecked through the body, as in the case of immunosuppressive diseases like AIDS, or attacks the body's own healthy cells, as in autoimmune diseases like multiple sclerosis and scleroderma.

The body fights intruders by two means, active and passive immunity. Both forms of immunity are necessary.

## Passive immunity

*Passive immunity* is protection by antibodies that a person receives from another human or animal. The most important form of passive immunity is the transfer of maternal antibodies during pregnancy. Some of the mother's antibodies, which pass to the developing fetus, can remain active in the baby for about a year after birth to protect the child from diseases such as measles and chickenpox.

Physicians use another form of passive immunity when they provide susceptible patients with concentrated antibodies that have been collected from donated blood. A person with a weakened immune system who has been exposed to chickenpox virus might receive an injection of chickenpox antibodies. A traveler preparing to leave for a country where hepatitis A virus is common may receive an injection of hepatitis A antibodies. A person who is bitten by a snake may even receive antibodies to the snake venom concentrated from the plasma of horses.

Passive immunity gives only short-term protection. When the antibodies transferred in this way lose their potency, the immune system is vulnerable once again.

## Active immunity

The active immune system is composed of two interacting and overlapping systems.

The *nonspecific immune system* consists of specialized cells, such as macrophages (literally "big eaters"), neutrophils, and natural killer cells as well as chemicals that send signals to cells. The nonspecific system acts within minutes or hours after viruses or bacteria infect the body. Its response to a second or third invasion of any particular germ is no greater or quicker than its response the first time.

The *specific immune system,* upon which vaccination depends, consists primarily of B lymphocytes, T lymphocytes, and antigen-presenting cells. The specific system takes several days and sometimes much longer to respond the first time a particular germ invades, but it responds more quickly and more powerfully the next time that germ invades. It does this by creating B and T *memory cells,* which stand ready for the next infection of the same antigen.

Some B lymphocytes become plasma cells, which in turn produce *antibodies.* These complex proteins circulate within the blood and lymph streams, attach to invading antigens, and mark them for destruction by other immune cells. Antibodies are quite specific: The antibodies for measles virus, for instance, will not interact with rubella virus (German measles), but they will interact with the measles *vaccine* virus.

## Vaccines and the active immune system

Vaccines are designed to work with the active immune system. When vaccines enter the body (most must be injected), the active immune system gears up for them, producing antibodies and memory cells. Because the vaccines resemble the corresponding germs (for example, the surface of the measles vaccine virus is very similar to the surface of the real measles virus), the system produces antibodies and memory cells that work against both the vaccine virus and, more importantly, against the actual virus. So when the real measles virus invades a vaccinated child, his immune system immediately identifies the virus and eliminates it before the child becomes ill.

## Two Main Types of Vaccines

### Live, attenuated vaccines

*Live vaccines* are made from live viruses that have been grown under special laboratory conditions so they are weakened, or *attenuated,* and thereby do not cause the symptoms or complications of the disease. But they do produce immunity, because the live vaccine virus displays the same special markers on its outer surface as the wild-type virus. When the live vaccine virus enters the body and begins replicating itself, the immune system jumps into action. Each component of the immune system does its part to process and destroy the antigen (or invader), and memory cells develop to guard against the next invasion of the disease.

The entire immune system responds to live vaccines as it does to infection from the wild-type disease. Thus, live injected vaccines usually require only one dose for lifelong immunity, just as one bout of measles or chickenpox will make most people immune for life.

Live vaccines, however, have several disadvantages. First, they usually require special storage and handling to keep them alive. Second, they could overwhelm a person who does not have a well-functioning immune system. This is why live vaccines should generally be withheld if a person has a weakened immune system.

Because of concern about the possibility that a live vaccine virus could harm a fetus, these vaccines are not given to pregnant women. Also, because antibodies passed from the mother to the fetus may interfere with live injected vaccines, these live vaccines are usually recommended at 12 months of age or later. (See Chapter 6 for more information on reasons to withhold vaccines.)

Because live vaccines are weak versions of the disease germs, they may cause a mild case of the disease they were designed to prevent. For example, chickenpox vaccination may cause a person to break out in a few pox or develop a low-grade fever. In real chickenpox a person usually develops 200 pox and substantial fever.

Live vaccines are used for the following diseases:

| | | | |
|---|---|---|---|
| Measles | Mumps | Rubella | Chickenpox |
| Polio (Oral) | Typhoid (Oral) | Tuberculosis | |
| Yellow Fever | Smallpox | | |

## Inactivated vaccines

*Inactivated vaccines* consist of whole microbes that have been killed by heat or chemicals (as in the inactivated polio vaccine, IPV) or are simply the important part of the microbe that provokes the immune system to respond (as in the hepatitis B vaccine). Unlike live vaccines, inactivated vaccines cannot replicate and so cannot cause even mild cases of the disease, but their presence still prompts the immune system to respond.

The inactivated vaccines cause a relatively weak response by the immune system, so usually the vaccination must be repeated. The advantages to inactivated vaccines include that they are not as fragile as live vaccines. Unlike live vaccines, inactivated vaccines are safe for persons who have weakened immune systems, for pregnant women, and for children under a year old. The side effects are generally just soreness where the vaccine was injected and possibly some fever shortly after vaccination.

Usually the outer coat of bacteria is made of protein, and the inactivated vaccines mimic this protein. Protein-based inactivated vaccines are used for the following diseases:

| | | | |
|---|---|---|---|
| Influenza | Polio (injected) | Pertussis | Plague |
| Hepatitis B | Hepatitis A | Lyme disease | |
| Rabies | Typhoid | Cholera | |

Some bacteria are literally sugarcoated. That is, their outer surface is composed of complex sugars, or *polysaccharides*. Vaccines against these bacteria must duplicate these special coats. Unfortunately, pure polysaccharide vaccines don't work well in infants and don't produce increasingly high antibody levels with subsequent doses. The meningococcal vaccine and the pneumococcal vaccine for older children and adults are pure polysaccharide vaccines.

A superior vaccine is produced by joining (conjugating) the polysaccharide to a protein. *Conjugate* vaccines are effective in infants and boost antibody levels with subsequent doses. The current Hib and the pneumococcal vaccine for infants and young children are conjugate polysaccharide vaccines.

*Toxoids* are another kind of inactivated vaccine. Instead of being made from killed germs, toxoids are made by inactivating the poisons, or toxins, produced by the germs. After you take the toxoid, your body is no better at fighting off infection to those germs, but it is much, much better at fighting off the effects of the germ's poison. The shots to prevent tetanus and diphtheria are toxoids.

## Vaccine Additives

Vaccines often contain antibiotics as well as preservatives to prevent bacteria from growing, stabilizers to maintain the vaccine's effectiveness, and adjuvants to stimulate production of antibodies. Although present only in minute amounts, these additives play an important role in vaccines. Some vaccine additives, such as thimerosal, aluminum, and formaldehyde, are controversial and are further discussed in Chapter 5.

### Antibiotics

Antibiotics prevent germs from growing in the vaccine cultures. Neomycin is commonly used, but penicillin and related antibiotics are not used in vaccines because many people are allergic to them.

### Preservatives

Vaccine vials that contain several doses need preservatives because each time a needle enters the vial there is a risk of contamination. Thimerosal is an extremely good preservative, but it is controversial because almost half of its contents is mercury, which is known to cause developmental problems in children when taken in large enough quantities. Formaldehyde, or formalin, is used to inactivate the polio vaccine virus in IPV and to kill germs in the cultures used to produce other vaccines.

### Stabilizers

Stabilizers maintain vaccine effectiveness despite heat, light, or other adverse conditions. Sulfites and monosodium glutamate (MSG), also found in many foods and alcoholic beverages, are used to stabilize some vaccines.

## Adjuvants

Aluminum, in the form of aluminum gels or salts of aluminum, is added to vaccines to help prompt antibodies to respond. For example, tetanus and diphtheria toxoids and pertussis vaccine are bound to aluminum salts.

## WHAT OTHER QUESTIONS DO PARENTS ASK?

*Q: Will too many shots overload my child's immune system?*

One parent observed that in the span of a few hours a North American child may eat her own nasal discharge, kiss the dog on the lips, taste the handrail at the airport, and still be able to survive quite nicely. The immune system is remarkably robust.

Careful and thorough studies done under the watchful eye of the FDA have shown that many vaccines can be given on the same day without a decrease in effectiveness or an increase in side effects. The same natural immune system that protects us from the multitude of personal microbiologic indiscretions of childhood is quite well equipped to protect us from a few vaccines.

*Q: Aren't some infectious diseases necessary to strengthen a child's immune system?*

No. If a person could go through life without a single infectious disease, his immune system would not have diminished. Exposure to deadly diseases like Hib, polio, pertussis and measles is not vital to a strong immune system!

*Q: Isn't disease just a natural part of life, while vaccines are unnatural and man-made?*

Yes, but by the same token, disease *and death* are a natural part of life. Because vaccines are man-made, they defy nature, but they also prolong the lives of infants, making infant mortality rates plummet and life expectancies soar.

*Q: Should I wait to vaccinate my child until he has recovered from being sick and his immune system is stronger?*

Your child's immune system is just as strong during most common minor illnesses as at other times, but he should not be given vaccines during a moderate to severe illness. This is because side effects of the vaccine (especially fever) may confuse the doctor regarding the course and management of the illness. Minor illnesses are not a reason to delay a vaccination.

*Q: Is the immune system down for a while after receiving a vaccine?*

A portion of your immune system (not the part that makes antibodies) may be depressed for as much as four weeks after live injected vaccines like measles, mumps, rubella, or chickenpox. You aren't more likely to get a serious infectious disease during those four weeks, but it is recommended that you hold off on getting another live, injected vaccine during that time.

*Q: A 4-month-old infant may receive five different vaccines (hepatitis B, Hib, polio, DTaP, pneumococcal) at one office visit. Is it safe to give so many vaccines at such a young age?*

The FDA tests vaccines that are given at the same time to be sure there is not an increase in side effects or a decrease in vaccine effectiveness. Each of the five vaccines has been tested in this way.

*Q: Aren't children naturally protected from these diseases by the immunity they get from their mothers? How long does this immunity last?*

Antibodies are passed from the mother to the fetus toward the end of pregnancy. These antibodies are an important source of protection from some diseases (such as measles), but not from others (such as polio). For full-term infants, these antibodies may last 6 to 18 months; the length of time varies. Severely premature infants are born without the mother's antibodies.

*Q: Won't the actual disease, versus the vaccine, give my daughter a higher antibody level, so her own children will have immunity longer?*

This is true for some but not all diseases. A mother's antibodies give good protection against some diseases (such as measles), but not others (such as polio).

If a girl gets measles, she will probably have a higher antibody level than girls whose antibody levels are a result of vaccination. When she is having children, she will pass along a greater amount of measles antibody, so her infant may be immune to measles longer than the infants of vaccinated mothers. This makes it more important to have an infant immunized with measles vaccine at 12 to 15 months of age.

Of course, a particular infant may have nonprotective antibody levels even if born to a woman who had the disease. Unless you do blood tests, it is impossible to be sure of an infant's immunity, so keep very young children away from anyone with measles, chickenpox, and so forth.

*Q: Won't the actual disease give my child lifelong immunity, whereas the vaccine will wear off?*

You can get some diseases—like tetanus—more than once, but once you have had most diseases you have lifelong immunity. You need to get some vaccines—like diphtheria and tetanus—periodically to stay completely protected, but you need only one injection of others (like measles vaccine) for lifelong immunity. In general, diseases are better at giving you lifelong immunity, but their disadvantage is that you might have to suffer through the disease and its complications (and possibly die) to become immune.

*Nothing can be done at once hastily and prudently.*
—Publilius Syrus, c. 42 B.C.

# Chapter 4

# How Vaccines Get Recommended

From the scientist's lab to your child's arm, vaccines go through a series of stages. It typically takes 15 years and an average of $500 million of manufacturers' money to get a new product from the laboratory to United States patients. Only about 5 out of 5,000 compounds that enter preclinical testing make it to trials involving humans, and only 1 of these 5 is ultimately approved for sale. Once the FDA licenses the vaccine for use, the CDC and medical organizations recommend who should receive it. The states then determine if the vaccine will be required for school entry. Some of the main organizations involved in the process are as follows.

- ✛ National Institutes of Health (NIH), a federal agency, conducts and funds other scientists to conduct biomedical research, including the development of vaccines.

- ✛ Food and Drug Administration (FDA), a federal agency, includes the Center for Biologics Evaluation and Research (CBER), which regulates all licensed and investigational vaccines used in the U.S. CBER ensures the safety, purity, potency, and effectiveness of vaccines. The center oversees the process of testing vaccines before and, to some extent, after they are licensed. The FDA grants manufacturers the product and manufacturing licenses.

When deciding whether or not to license a vaccine, the manufacturer and the FDA present their findings to the Vaccines and Related Biological Products Advisory Committee (VRBPAC), typically at an open, public forum. VRBPAC is composed of prominent scientists and physicians from academia and senior officials from government agencies. VRBPAC membership is supplemented with three or more persons who have special expertise in the particular vaccine at issue. The FDA is not required to follow the advice or recommendations of VRBPAC, but it usually does.

✛ Centers for Disease Control and Prevention (CDC), a federal agency, includes the National Immunization Program, which is responsible for tasks that range from monitoring reports of childhood vaccine-preventable diseases, to evaluating vaccine safety after licensure, to helping with worldwide eradication of polio. The CDC also includes the National Vaccine Program, which coordinates the vaccine efforts of many federal agencies, and the National Center for Infectious Diseases which, among many other tasks, leads CDC's efforts to reduce the incidence of infectious hepatitis and meningococcus.

The Advisory Committee on Immunization Practices (ACIP) provides guidance regarding the use of vaccines and other biologic products (such as immune globulin) to the U.S. Secretary and Assistant Secretary for Health and to CDC's director. ACIP meets three times a year in an open, public forum. It is made up of 12 members who are leaders in vaccine research and public health. The committee is assisted by nonvoting, ex officio members from federal agencies and medical organizations and by topic specialists.

After the ACIP makes vaccine recommendations, CDC decides whether or not to accept them. CDC publishes its vaccination recommendations, as well as articles on infectious diseases and other public health concerns, in its weekly publication *Morbidity and Mortality Weekly (MMWR)*.

⊕ Several medical organizations participate in the development of national vaccine policy, but two organizations are particularly important to childhood immunization. The American Academy of Pediatrics (AAP) is a private professional organization of physicians who specialize in pediatrics. The AAP has a prestigious 12-member standing committee—the Committee on Infectious Diseases (COID)—composed of pediatric infectious disease subspecialists who recommend immunization policy to the chief executive body of the AAP. The report of the COID is published periodically in a volume called the "Red Book."

The American Academy of Family Physicians (AAFP) is a private professional organization of family physicians. Like AAP, AAFP sends a representative to serve on ACIP and issues its own recommendations on childhood and adult vaccines.

## THE PROCESS FROM TESTING TO RECOMMENDATION

### What tests do vaccines undergo before they are licensed?

Vaccines must pass a series of tests before being licensed. Safety tests in animals must be passed before the three phases of testing in humans, called clinical trials, can be initiated. The manufacturer who wishes to begin clinical trials with a vaccine must submit an Investigational New Drug Application to FDA describing vaccine components, methods of manufacture, and methods to ensure quality control. Vaccine clinical trials are then usually done in three phases.

1. In Phase 1, the initial testing in humans, a series of brief studies are conducted in small numbers of adults (usually fewer than 20). The studies are repeated in groups of progressively younger patients. Though safety is the prime concern at this stage, scientists also evaluate the immune system's response to the vaccine and try to determine the optimal dose.

2. In Phase 2, 50 to several hundred volunteers are vaccinated. In addition to evaluating safety and immune response, Phase 2 studies begin to look at how well the vaccine protects people under optimal circumstances.

3. In Phase 3, the final phase before licensure, anywhere from 1,000 to 100,000—but most typically about 10,000—human volunteers are vaccinated and monitored for a year or two at most. Safety and protection from disease are the focus. The size of these studies depends on several factors. For example, the studies are smaller if no other vaccine is available or if the target disease is very common.

Following successful completion of all three phases of clinical testing, the manufacturer usually submits a Biologics License Application. This must provide the FDA review team with sufficient information on the safety and efficacy of the product to allow for a risk-benefit assessment in the vaccine's intended population. Also at this time, the proposed manufacturing facility will have a pre-approval inspection. A single violation of good manufacturing practices will cause the license to be delayed.

### How do licensed vaccines become recommended?

Though they attempt to coordinate, AAP, AAFP, and CDC each formulate separate vaccination recommendations. Their recommendations address questions such as, "What groups of people should receive this vaccine?" and "What is the optimal schedule for vaccination?" The distribution of the infection and its complications, as well as vaccine safety and effectiveness, must each be considered.

Economists are asked to estimate the costs and savings generated by a vaccination program, and these data are also considered. The Vaccines for Children Program, created by Congress, provides vaccines for children who have limited or no insurance, but it only covers vaccines that CDC recommends universally. ACIP members realize that a vote to recommend a childhood vaccine universally means that not only will insurance companies be asked to pay millions of dollars to cover this vaccine, but also the U.S. government will obliged to pay millions of tax dollars for it each year.

### How do recommended vaccines become required for school entry?

There are no national immunization laws. However, before a child is permitted to attend school, all states require evidence of vaccination against diphtheria, measles, rubella, and polio, and most states also require tetanus, pertussis, and mumps vaccination. (See Figure 4-1 for a list of vaccine requirements by state.) All states allow exemptions from these school entry laws under certain circumstances. See Chapter 7 for details on these state laws and exemptions.

## POST-RECOMMENDATION REVIEW

### What vaccine monitoring is done after licensure?

What if a serious side effect is rare, occurring only in 1 out of 40,000 children? The prelicensure testing, which may have included only 10,000 children, probably would not have detected it. After the vaccine is licensed and given to 4 million children every year, on average each year 100 children would develop the side effect. With this example in mind, how can we know enough to feel safe using a vaccine until a few million people have taken it? Yet how can we expect a vaccine to be tested in millions of children before it is licensed?

The FDA, CDC, and vaccine manufacturers are responsible for vaccine research and surveillance *after* licensure to evaluate

1. The occurrence of rare side effects;

2. The safety and efficacy of the vaccine in populations not sufficiently represented during Phase 3 studies, such as the elderly and those with chronic illness; and

3. The vaccine's long-term effectiveness.

In 1990, CDC established the Vaccine Safety Datalink (VSD) to evaluate possible vaccine side effects. VSD links information about vaccination, hospitalization, and medical records for members of four large managed care groups that serve about 2 percent of the U.S. population in the relevant age groups.

Also in 1990, CDC and FDA started the Vaccine Adverse Event Reporting System (VAERS) to keep a closer surveillance of vaccines after licensure. (See Figure 4-2 for a sample VAERS reporting form.) Patients, their families, and healthcare professionals can report any condition they suspect a vaccine may have caused, and vaccine manufacturers are *required* to report

Figure 4-1

# IMMUNIZATION REQUIREMENTS BY STATE, 1999–2000

| STATE | Diphtheria | Tetanus | Pertussis* | Measles | Mumps | Rubella | Hepatitis A | Hepatitis B | Chickenpox | Polio |
|---|---|---|---|---|---|---|---|---|---|---|
| Alabama | X | X | X | X | X | X | | | | X |
| Alaska | X | X | X | X | X | X | | | | X |
| Arizona | X | X | X | X | X | X | | K-1 | | X |
| Arkansas | X | X | X | X | | X | | | | X |
| California | X | X | X | X | X | X | | | | X |
| Colorado | X | X | X | X | X | X | | ≥18 mo, K-1, 7-8 | ≥18 mo | X |
| Connecticut | X | X | X | X | X | X | | X | | X |
| Delaware | X | X | X | X | X | X | | | | X |
| Dist. of Col. | X | X | X | X | X | X | | K | Daycare, K-9 | X |
| Florida | X | X | X | X | X | X | | K, 7-8 | | X |
| Georgia | X | X | X | X | X | X | | K | | X |
| Hawaii | X | X | X | X | X | X | | X | | X |
| Idaho | X | X | | X | X | X | | X | | X |
| Illinois | X | X | X | X | X | X | | 5 | | X |
| Indiana | X | X | X | X | X | X | | X | | X |
| Iowa | X | X | X | X | | X | | K | | X |
| Kansas | X | X | X | X | X | X | | | | X |
| Kentucky | X | X | X | X | X | X | | X | | X |
| Louisiana | New Entrants | New Entrants | New Entrants | New Entrants | New Entrants | New Entrants | | K | | New Entrants |
| Maine | X | X | | X | X | X | | | | X |
| Maryland | X | X | X | X | X | X | | | Daycare | X |
| Massachusetts | X | X | X | X | X | X | | K-2 | Daycare, K, 7 | X |
| Michigan | New Entrants | New Entrants | New Entrants | New Entrants | New Entrants | New Entrants | | | Daycare, New entrants | New Entrants |
| Minnesota | X | X | X | X | X | X | | | | X |
| Mississippi | X | X | X | X | X | X | | | | X |
| Missouri | X | X | X | X | X | X | | K-1 | | X |
| Montana | X | X | X | X | X | X | | | | X |
| Nebraska | X | X | X | X | X | X | | | | X |
| Nevada | X | X | X | X | X | X | | | | X |
| New Hampshire | X | X | X | X | X | X | | X | | X |
| New Jersey | X | X | X | X | X | X | | | | X |
| New Mexico | X | X | X | X | X | X | | | | X |
| New York | X | | | X | X | X | | X | | X |
| North Carolina | X | X | X | X | X | X | | X | | X |
| North Dakota | X | X | X | X | X | X | | | | X |
| Ohio | X | X | X | X | X | X | | | | X |
| Oklahoma | X | X | X | X | K-11 | X | K, 7 | K, 7-8 | Daycare, K | X |
| Oregon | X | X | | X | X | X | | K | Daycare, K, 7 | X |
| Pennsylvania | X | X | | X | X | X | | K | | X |
| Puerto Rico | X | X | X | X | X | X | | K-1, 7-8 | | X |
| Rhode Island | X | X | X | X | X | X | | | Daycare, K, 1, 7 | X |
| South Carolina | New Entrants | New Entrants | New Entrants | X | X | X | | K, 1, 7 | | X |
| South Dakota | X | X | X | X | X | X | | | | X |
| Tennessee | X | X | X | X | X | X | | K | Daycare | X |
| Texas | X | X | | X | X | X | | X | Daycare, K, Middle school | X |
| Utah | X | X | X | X | X | X | | K | | X |
| Vermont | X | X | X | X | | X | | | Daycare | X |
| Virginia | X | X | X | X | X | X | | K | Daycare | X |
| Washington | X | X | X | X | X | X | | K-1 | | X |
| West Virginia | New Entrants | New Entrants | New Entrants | X | | X | | | | New Entrants |
| Wisconsin | X | X | X | X | X | X | | K-1, 7, 8 | | X |
| Wyoming | X | X | X | X | X | X | | 7 | | X |

*Source:* State Immunization Requirements 1998–1999, *p. 1*

**Figure 4-2**

# VAERS REPORTING FORM

---

**VACCINE ADVERSE EVENT REPORTING SYSTEM**
24 Hour Toll Free Information 1-800-822-7967
P.O. Box 1100, Rockville, MD 20849-1100
**VAERS**
**PATIENT IDENTITY KEPT CONFIDENTIAL**

**For CDC/FDA Use Only**
VAERS Number _____

Date Received _____

Patient Name:

Vaccine administered by (Name): _____

Form completed by (Name): _____

Last          First          M.I.

Responsible
Physician _____
Facility Name/Address

Relation      ☐ Vaccine Provider  ☐ Patient/Parent
to Patient    ☐ Manufacturer       ☐ Other
Address (if different from patient or provider)

Address

City          State    Zip
Telephone no. (___) _____

City          State    Zip
Telephone no. (___) _____

City          State    Zip
Telephone no. (___) _____

| 1. State | 2. County where administered | 3. Date of birth mm / dd / yy | 4. Patient age | 5. Sex ☐M ☐F | 6. Date form completed mm / dd / yy |

7. Describe adverse events(s) (symptoms, signs, time course) and treatment, if any

8. Check all appropriate:
☐ Patient died      (date ___ / ___ / ___)
☐ Life threatening illness
☐ Required emergency room/doctor visit
☐ Required hospitalization (_____days)
☐ Resulted in prolongation of hospitalization
☐ Resulted in permanent disability
☐ None of the above

9. Patient recovered    ☐YES  ☐NO  ☐UNKNOWN

10. Date of vaccination    11. Adverse event onset

12. Relevant diagnostic tests/laboratory data

___ / ___ / ___ mm dd yy AM    ___ / ___ / ___ mm dd yy AM
Time _____ PM  Time _____ PM

13. Enter all vaccines given on date listed in no. 10

| Vaccine (type) | Manufacturer | Lot number | Route/Site | No. Previous Doses |
|---|---|---|---|---|
| a. | | | | |
| b. | | | | |
| c. | | | | |
| d. | | | | |

14. Any other vaccinations within 4 weeks prior to the date listed in no. 10

| Vaccine (type) | Manufacturer | Lot number | Route/Site | No. Previous doses | Date given |
|---|---|---|---|---|---|
| a. | | | | | |
| b. | | | | | |

15. Vaccinated at:
☐ Private doctor's office/hospital   ☐ Military clinic/hospital
☐ Public health clinic/hospital      ☐ Other/unknown

16. Vaccine purchased with:
☐ Private funds   ☐ Military funds
☐ Public funds    ☐ Other/unknown

17. Other medications

18. Illness at time of vaccination (specify)

19. Pre-existing physician-diagnosed allergies, birth defects, medial conditions(specify)

20. Have you reported this adverse event previously?    ☐ No    ☐ To health department
☐ To doctor    ☐ To manufacturer

**Only for children 5 and under**
22. Birth weight _____ lb. _____ oz.
23. No. of brother and sisters

21. Adverse event following prior vaccination (check all applicable, specify)

| | Adverse Event | Onset Age | Type Vaccine | Dose no. in series |
|---|---|---|---|---|
| ☐In patient | | | | |
| ☐In brother or sister | | | | |

**Only for reports submitted by manufacturer/immunization project**
24. Mfr./imm. proj. report no.
25. Date received by mfr./imm.proj.

26. 15 day report?    ☐ Yes  ☐ No
27. Report type    ☐ Initial  ☐ Follow-Up

Health care providers and manufacturers are required by law (42 USC 300aa-25) to report reactions to vaccines listed in the Table of Reportable Events Following Immunization Reports for reactions to other vaccines are voluntary except when required as a condition of immunization grant awards.

Form VAERS-1(FDA)

*Note: To obtain copies of the VAERS form or to get assistance in filling out the form, call 800-822-7967, or download the form from http://www.fda.gov/cber/vaers.*

side effects they hear about. VAERS can be used to determine if reports of possible vaccine side effects are clustering in certain areas of the country (which might indicate a problem with a vaccine lot) or at a set interval after the vaccine (which might indicate a problem with the vaccine itself).

### What is a recent example of a vaccine being re-examined?

Several cases of bowel obstruction following vaccination for rotavirus were reported to VAERS. The timing of these cases tipped off a medical officer at the CDC National Immunization Program that a problem existed with the rotavirus vaccine. The number of cases reported to VAERS was higher than expected, and they clustered in the week following rotavirus vaccination. What Dr. Chuck Vitek saw in that VAERS report led to a full-blown scientific investigation and, eventually, to the removal of the vaccine from the U.S. market.

Rotavirus vaccine was created to prevent the most common form of serious infant diarrhea. In the U.S. each year it kills 20 to 40 people and results in 50,000 hospitalizations, mostly of children under age 3. In prelicensure studies, 5 out of 10,000 (0.05 percent) of the vaccine recipients and 1 out of 4,600 (0.02 percent) of the placebo recipients developed bowel obstruction (in the form of intussusception); no significant difference appeared to exist between the groups. The ACIP was quite excited about the prospect of preventing this major infectious disease and so at their March 1998 meeting the members voted to recommend rotavirus vaccine for all infants, even *before* the first rotavirus vaccine was licensed in the U.S. (which occurred in August 1998).

Between September 1998 and June 1999, approximately 1.5 million doses of rotavirus vaccine were given to young children. By July 7, 1999, VAERS received 15 reports of intussusception following rotavirus vaccination, 80 percent within 7 days of vaccination. Only 3 cases would be expected to be reported for that many children. Was the vaccine actually causing the intussusceptions?

In the summer of 1999 the CDC began an intensive, large study of the problem and published, in conjunction with the American Academy of Pediatrics, a recommendation to postpone use of the rotavirus vaccine until definitive data were available. By October 1999, sufficient data had accumulated to implicate rotavirus vaccine as the cause for the intussusception cases, so CDC and the medical organizations rescinded their recommendation and the manufacturer withdrew the vaccine from the market. This was the first vaccine in over two decades to have been recalled because of safety concerns.

## How can the U.S. improve the vaccine approval process?

The rotavirus vaccine story demonstrates the strength of the postlicensure surveillance system, but it raises questions about the approval process. What lessons can we learn from this incident?

**Time pressures.** A persistent tension exists between thoroughness and speediness. The FDA is under significant pressure by the pharmaceutical industry, Congress, and consumers to approve new drugs more rapidly than in years past. The FDA is charged with making sure the pharmaceutical industry delivers safe, pure, potent, and effective vaccines to prevent important diseases. But their job is also to make these vaccines available to the American public as soon as possible. Though it is rare for a licensed vaccine (like rotavirus) to be found to have side effects that tip the benefit-risk balance, critics wonder if the licensure system moves too quickly and approvals come too easily.

The same question has been asked of the ACIP vaccine recommendation process. Should there be a delay before new vaccines are recommended for all children? That would allow a postlicensure surveillance period to uncover rare side effects, but the delay would also leave children exposed for a longer time to the given disease. Do we as parents want to risk that delay?

**ACIP composition.** Specialists in pediatric infectious diseases are usually researchers who obtain research grants from governmental sources, foundations, and pharmaceutical companies. Pharmaceutical companies also ask them for consultation from time to time. To avoid conflicts of interest, ACIP members must abstain from voting if they have received grant money or consultation fees from a manufacturer whose profits would be affected by the decision. During 1999, 10 of the 12 board members had a conflict of interest with at least one vaccine manufacturer; one board member had a conflict with every major vaccine manufacturer. So due to conflicts of interest, only a fraction of ACIP board members were able to vote on any particular vaccine issue before them. Is it possible to assemble a panel with as much expertise but fewer conflicts of interest?

**Complete information.** In some instances, not all the information that exists about a vaccine is available to the advisory boards. Sometimes the information is proprietary: Vaccine manufacturers have the legal right not to share it for reasons of competition. Sometimes the information is overlooked. For example, a *Wall Street Journal* story described a 1989 study of an earlier rotavirus vaccine made by a French manufacturer and tested in China in which 2 cases of intussusception were found among 351 vaccinated infants, but neither the FDA nor CDC advisory boards were aware of the study when making their recommendations. How can we make sure that the advisory boards have all the data about a vaccine so they can make a fully informed decision?

## CONCLUSION

According to Dr. David Satcher, the U.S. Surgeon General, our "stringent regulation process for licensing vaccines...serves as a model for all countries." The process by which licensed vaccines are recommended is independent and guided by some of the best scientists in the country. The result is a remarkable U.S. vaccine safety record, with some notable exceptions. While acknowledging that the system is not perfect, Dr. Peter Patriarca, Director of the Viral Products Center for Biologics Evaluation and Research for the FDA, assures parents: "I think the vaccine approval process is quite sound, and the American public, including parents, should not get overly concerned."

*If a little knowledge is dangerous, where is the man who has so much as to be out of danger?*

—Thomas Huxley

# Chapter 5

# Vaccine Controversies

When the news media gives vaccine controversies much attention, we parents are faced with the difficult task of separating worrisome conjecture from facts meriting a change in how we vaccinate our children. This task is no less difficult for the scientists who dedicate themselves to it.

Historical examples show that problems with vaccines in the past have led to changes in the U.S. immunization program. Vaccine controversies today may lead to more changes, but they are certainly driving a notable increase in the search for rare adverse effects. Sensitive new lab techniques are being used, for example, to look for measles virus genes in the gut cells of children with inflammatory bowel disease. Powerful information systems are in place to gather and rapidly analyze reports of vaccine side effects and to make the data available to the public.

## CURRENT CONTROVERSIES: VACCINATION AND CHRONIC ILLNESS

*The increasing incidence of diabetes, autism, and other medical conditions for which no specific etiology has been identified parallels the increase in many other factors such as the use of wireless communications, computers, and fast food restaurants. One could easily hypothesize that these factors or many other changes in our lifestyles contributed to the increases in these diseases, but there is no scientific evidence to support these ideas.*

—Dr. Neal Halsey,
Director of the Institute for Vaccine Safety
Johns Hopkins University School of Public Health

The topics below address some of the more common concerns repeated in news stories. For discussions of notable historical controversies, see Chapter 4 on the rotavirus vaccine, Chapter 10 on polio for the issues of SV40 and the Cutter vaccine, and Chapter 16 on influenza for the swine flu.

## Asthma

Studies have shown an increase in the prevalence of asthma in recent years. Research supports the roles of air pollution and cigarette smoke in this increase. The Wellington Asthma Research Group (WARG) has implicated vaccines, as well. They hypothesize that children in the developed world are now less likely to develop certain infections in early infancy, which then allows their immune system to be more prone to developing allergic sensitization. However, a British study of 9,444 children found no association between immunization and wheezing from asthma.

## Autism

Since the 1980s, both the United States and Britain have seen dramatic increases in the number of children diagnosed with autism, a disorder of communication, social cognition, and sensory integration. In California the number of young children diagnosed with autism increased 273 percent between 1987 and 1998, while other developmental disorders showed increases of 47 percent or less.

Autism is often diagnosed just after a child is expected to begin talking at about 18 months of age, which is also shortly after MMR is usually given. Some parent groups say they noticed the dramatic increase in autism cases in California after 1978, when the combination vaccine MMR was added to the school entry requirements. They point out that previously, the measles, mumps, and rubella vaccines were given separately at different times during early childhood.

In response to these concerns, the National Institutes of Health assembled in 1996 a working group on autism. They described anatomic differences in the brains of autistics as being "consistent with a developmental curtailment that takes place at some point earlier than 30 weeks gestation"—that is, before birth. Such differences would preclude vaccination as a possible cause.

Then, in 1999, *Lancet* published a British study of 498 autistic children. The study revealed that the number of children diagnosed with autism rose each year from 1979 to 1992, and that no evidence showed a sudden increase of cases in 1987, the first year MMR was introduced. The authors concluded that MMR did not appear to cause autism.

Additional studies are underway to seek the cause of autism.

## Guillain-Barré Syndrome (GBS)

GBS is a rare disorder of the nervous system that causes temporary paralysis and loss of reflexes. The muscle weakness usually begins in the legs and moves to the arms. Most patients recover, but up to 6 percent of persons with GBS die from complications. No one knows what causes GBS, but a virus is suspected because GBS is often preceded by an infectious illness. A 1998 CDC study suggested the 1992–93 and 1993–94 influenza vaccines may have increased the rate of GBS by 1 case per million vaccinations, but it is difficult to be certain of the precise increase with such rare events. ACIP suggests that, while avoiding future influenza vaccinations may be prudent for persons who developed GBS within six weeks of a previous influenza vaccination, for those at high risk for severe complications from influenza, the benefits of vaccination justify the risks. The National Injury Compensation Program does not cover GBS after flu vaccine, but assistance or compensation may be available through the Social Security Administration or a state assistance program.

No evidence suggests an increased risk of GBS after routine childhood vaccines.

## Diabetes

While most diabetes develops in middle age when the cells of the body become resistant to insulin, in 5 to 10 percent of diabetes, the pancreas cannot produce insulin. This is called Type I diabetes. Without insulin, the cells cannot use glucose, so sugar builds up in the bloodstream and spills into the urine. Symptoms of diabetes include excessive urination, thirst, hunger, dehydration, and weight loss. Insulin injections must be taken daily to keep blood glucose levels stable. Uncontrolled diabetes can lead to blindness, loss of hearing, heart and kidney disease, strokes, cataracts, nerve damage, paralysis of the intestinal tract, gangrene requiring amputation of limbs, and death.

The claims and evidence associating vaccines and diabetes include the following:

✛ Babies infected with the natural rubella virus in their mother's womb may be born with congenital rubella syndrome, which is associated with Type I diabetes. Similarly, natural mumps disease has been associated with Type I diabetes. But no researcher has found a link between diabetes and the vaccine rubella virus or vaccine mumps virus used in the U.S., which are very much weaker than the natural viruses.

Among rats that have been genetically altered to be particularly prone to diabetes, many stimuli to the immune system—including vaccination—increase the frequency of diabetes, but it is a long stretch to extrapolate from these rodents to human babies.

✛ A 1997 study compared countries that used different immunization schedules. The team reported that immunization at birth with the tuberculosis vaccine reduced the incidence of diabetes, whereas giving the vaccine after 2 months of age increased the incidence. Of course, they could not take into account all the differences between the countries' racial compositions and environmental factors.

Dr. Bart Classen also suggested that additional doses of Hib vaccine cause diabetes. He analyzed other researchers' data from

Finland and found that within a 10-year follow-up period, 205 children who received four doses of Hib vaccine developed diabetes, but only 185 children who received one dose of Hib vaccine developed diabetes. However, to compare these two numbers statistically, we must know how many children were in each follow-up group. The Finnish investigators themselves have refuted Dr. Classen's claim.

In 1995, the National Institutes of Health convened an expert panel to evaluate the data linking diabetes and vaccination. Again in 1998, the National Institutes of Allergy and Infectious Diseases organized a meeting of public and private organizations to review what was known on the subject. Both panels concluded that human studies do not indicate a link between diabetes and either vaccination or the timing of vaccination. Because autoimmune antibodies (that is, antibodies that attack one's own cells) may be a cause of Type I diabetes, in 1999, the Diabetes Autoimmunity Study in the Young examined 317 children who had first-degree relatives with Type I diabetes. They found no difference in vaccination status between the group of children who developed autoimmune antibodies and those who did not.

## Multiple Sclerosis (MS)

In MS the immune system attacks and damages the fatty material surrounding nerves in the brain and spinal cord. The fatty material, or myelin, serves to facilitate conduction of nerve signals; damage to the myelin—or demyelination—disrupts the signals. The area of the brain or spinal cord affected determines what symptoms result. Though the cause of MS is still unknown, it is likely to be both genetic and environmental. It is most common in young adult females, especially those in northern latitudes.

Between 1990 and the summer of 1999, 76 cases of MS following vaccination for hepatitis B were reported to the Vaccine Adverse Event Reporting System. Two expert panels reviewed all available data on hepatitis B vaccine's relationship with MS and other demyelinating disorders, but they could find no scientific basis for the allegations. The National Multiple Sclerosis Society, the World Health Organization, and the European Viral

Hepatitis Prevention Board concur that no current evidence links hepatitis B vaccination and multiple sclerosis.

### Sudden Infant Death Syndrome (SIDS)

SIDS, or crib death, has been reported after vaccination. DTP and hepatitis B vaccines have been singled out for investigation, but current evidence supports continued vaccination. One study showed that children who received the DTP vaccine were actually less likely to die of SIDS than unvaccinated infants. Similarly, the number of cases of SIDS in the U.S. dropped during the same years when the number of infants receiving hepatitis B vaccine increased. The drop in SIDS is probably not due to the vaccine but to Back to Sleep, a program that encourages parents to put infants on their backs rather than their stomachs when sleeping. Nonetheless, the drop in SIDS deaths at a time when millions more infants were being vaccinated against hepatitis B is reassuring.

## THE NUMBER OF VACCINES

Current concerns about vaccination may be fueled, in part, by the sheer number of recommended vaccines. The number of vaccines that children receive has increased steadily, as has protection against infectious diseases. While many are grateful for the additional vaccines, they dread the extra injections and look to more combination vaccines and to new needle-free forms of immunization. Others, willing to forego protection against some diseases, are calling for fewer vaccines overall.

ACIP is giving serious consideration to the necessity for each dose of each vaccine. For example, the question was raised at the October 1999 ACIP meeting if, with the world on the brink of polio eradication, the U.S. could safely go to a three-dose IPV series (the series currently includes a fourth dose booster).

Some argue that the number of vaccines for children should be reduced because the vaccines might overload children's immune systems. However, the immune system is remarkably powerful, and vaccines are child's play compared to the infectious load presented by the natural world. Children are exposed to many thousands of germs beginning at the moment of birth.

Further, each bacterium contains hundreds of parts—proteins, sugars, fats, DNA, and RNA—which the immune system must respond to. In fact, according to Dr. Neal Halsey a single bout of strep throat results in immune responses to 25 to 50 different substances.

## VACCINE ADDITIVES AND CONTAMINANTS

Vaccines contain *additives* such as preservatives and antibiotics (see page 20). These are included in minute quantities, but they must be monitored for safety. The FDA also requires manufacturers to have procedures to detect and prevent the inclusion of vaccine *contaminants*, such as unwanted viruses and bacteria. For example, when the polio vaccines are produced, the manufacturers are required to test cell lines used for the production of the vaccine for many infectious agents such as tuberculosis, SV40, herpes viruses, and Coxsackie virus. In the future the FDA may require still more safety measures to make sure vaccines do not contain contaminants.

### Thimerosal

In 1999 the FDA announced that the recommended childhood vaccines contain more thimerosal—a preservative that is about half mercury—than may be safe. In large quantities mercury can cause brain damage. A good deal of controversy arose over the issue because three different U.S. agencies have three different permissible levels, and only the one from the Environmental Protection Agency was exceeded. Additionally, the established levels relate to ongoing daily exposure to a compound questionably related to thimerosal, so no one was sure how to extrapolate to thimerosal in vaccines. Nonetheless, because there was reasonable uncertainty, the U.S. Public Health Service and the American Academy of Pediatrics asked vaccine manufacturers to eliminate thimerosal from vaccines. At least one brand of every vaccine does not contain thimerosal as a preservative, and it is likely that thimerosal will be out of almost all childhood vaccines soon.

### Aluminum

Aluminum gels or salts are in vaccines to help stimulate the production of antibodies. The World Health Organization reported that deposits of aluminum had been found in certain white blood cells in muscles where vaccines had been given. This was first recognized in 1993 and has almost exclusively been reported in France. The significance of the finding is unknown.

### Human Immunodeficiency Virus (HIV)

In his book *The River: A Journey to the Source of HIV and AIDS,* British journalist Edward Hooper hypothesizes that the AIDS virus originally passed from chimpanzees to humans in the late 1950s during the early testing of oral polio vaccine (OPV) in the Congo. However, the physicians who conducted the implicated trials point out that they never used chimpanzee tissues to produce the polio vaccine; they used chimpanzees for *testing* the vaccine. The scientists also note that the crossover of HIV from chimpanzees into humans probably occurred before polio vaccine was used in the Congo. In November 1999, the research institute that developed the OPV vaccine announced that, to reach a definitive conclusion, it would allow two independent laboratories to test both of the original vaccine lots.

## CONCLUSION

In the best of all worlds, there would be no controversies over the safety of vaccines; all vaccines would be 100 percent safe and 100 percent effective. Until that day, as Dr. Neal Halsey pointed out in his testimony before the U.S. House of Representatives Committee on Government Reform in October 1999, "Vaccine safety should be based on good science, not hypotheses, opinion, individual beliefs, or observations. Federal agencies responsible for vaccine safety and major universities have procedures to assure high-quality scientific research and reviews of vaccine safety issues." It is Congress's role, he stated, to "be concerned about vaccine safety" and to "provide sufficient resources to assure that the best possible science is conducted to assist with the development of vaccine policy."

*The scars of others should teach us caution.*

—St. Jerome

# Chapter 6

# Medical Reasons Not to Vaccinate

Going through life without vaccinations may be hazardous to your health, but not everyone should be vaccinated. One person's immune system may overreact to a particular vaccine, whereas another person's may not mount enough of a response. A simple screening sheet (Figure 6-1) highlights medical reasons for not being vaccinated. Although children with the following conditions should avoid or delay vaccination, disease outbreaks in the community might cause parents and physicians to reconsider a childhood vaccine.

## ALLERGIES

### Severe allergic reactions to a vaccine

If your child had a severe allergic reaction (for instance, immediate hives, difficulty breathing, shock) after a vaccine, you should not accept that particular vaccine again. Your child may need to see an allergist to sort out which vaccine caused the allergic reaction. Also, if he or she has a severe allergy to any of the ingredients in a vaccine, your child should not be given that particular vaccine. Severe allergic reactions can cause hives to break out,

**Figure 6-1**
## VACCINATION SCREENING FORM

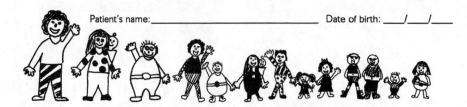

Patient's name: _____ Date of birth: ____/____/____

# Screening Questionnaire
# for Child and Teen Immunization

**For parents/guardians:** The following questions will help us determine which vaccines may be given in clinic today. Please answer these questions by checking the boxes. If the question is not clear, please ask the nurse or doctor to explain it.

|  | Yes | No | Don't Know |
|---|---|---|---|
| 1. Is the child sick today? | ☐ | ☐ | ☐ |
| 2. Does the child have allergies to medications, food, or any vaccine? | ☐ | ☐ | ☐ |
| 3. Has the child had a serious reaction to a vaccine in the past? | ☐ | ☐ | ☐ |
| 4. Has the child had a seizure or a brain problem? | ☐ | ☐ | ☐ |
| 5. Does the child, or any person who lives with or takes care of the child, have cancer, leukemia, AIDS, or any other immune system problem? | ☐ | ☐ | ☐ |
| 6. Has the child, or any person who lives with or takes care of the child, taken cortisone, prednisone, other steroids, anticancer drugs, or x-ray treatments in the past 3 months? | ☐ | ☐ | ☐ |
| 7. Has the child received a transfusion of blood or plasma, or been given a medicine called immune (gamma) globulin in the past year? | ☐ | ☐ | ☐ |
| 8. Is the child/teen pregnant or is there a chance she could become pregnant in the next three months? | ☐ | ☐ | ☐ |

Parent/guardian signature: _____ Date : _____

**Did you bring your child's immunization record card with you?**  yes ☐   no ☐

It is important for you to have a personal record of your child's shots. If you don't have a record card, ask the child's doctor or nurse to give you one! Bring this record with you every time you bring your child to the clinic. Make sure your clinic records all your child's vaccinations on it. Your child will need this card to enter daycare, kindergarten, junior high, etc.

Item #P4060 (8/99)

Immunization Action Coalition • 1573 Selby Avenue • St. Paul, MN 55104 • (651) 647-9009 • www.immunize.org

can prompt a person's airway to swell to the point that breathing becomes severely or completely obstructed, and can send a person into shock.

Table 6-1 lists the ingredients in each vaccine that are the most common allergy triggers. Note that no U.S. vaccine contains any penicillin or penicillin-related antibiotics (such as amoxicillin or cephalosporins).

Many persons have *local* allergic reactions to certain medicines, developing an irritation where the medicine has been applied—such as getting red eyes if they use an eye ointment with neomycin or a contact lens solution with thimerosal (see Chapter 5) in it. These local reactions are totally different from the life-threatening allergies that would prevent a person from being vaccinated. They are generally limited to the specific location and are short-lived.

## Common allergens and vaccines

Common allergies that people have to dust, pollen, milk, or animals do not affect vaccination. The exception would be to chicken eggs; if anyone in your family is severely allergic to these, then he or she should not receive the injected flu vaccine. Duck proteins, another common allergen, are not in U.S. vaccines.

**Table 6-1**
## VACCINE INGREDIENTS THAT ARE ALLERGY TRIGGERS

| Vaccine | Vaccine ingredient as allergy trigger |
|---|---|
| Hepatitis B | Baker's yeast |
| DTaP | — |
| IPV (polio) | Neomycin, streptomycin, polymyxin B (antibiotics) |
| Hib | — |
| MMR | Gelatin, neomycin |
| Chickenpox | Gelatin, neomycin |
| Hepatitis A | — |
| Pneumococcus | — |
| Flu | Chicken eggs; a tiny amount of neomycin (an antibiotic, about as much as in a skin test for allergy) |

## ENCEPHALITIS

Encephalitis, an inflammation of the brain, is a severe condition that requires hospitalization for symptoms that may range from confusion to coma. If your child develops encephalitis within seven days after receiving DTaP, then he or she should definitely not receive more doses of that vaccine.

## MODERATE TO SEVERE ILLNESS AT THE TIME OF VACCINATION

If your child is ill when it is time for his or her vaccination, then consult the healthcare giver. You might need to postpone the vaccination.

Generally, minor illnesses—such as a cold, an earache, or diarrhea—are not a good reason to postpone vaccination. For instance, if the doctor examines your feverish child and finds she has an ear infection, then giving her vaccines at the same time as the antibiotics for the ear infection is completely acceptable. Vaccines can be given at the same time as antibiotics and medicine to reduce fever. The vaccines work just as well, and there is no increase in vaccine side effects.

Moderate to severe illness, however, is a good reason to postpone vaccination. The side effects of the vaccine may confuse the doctor about how the illness is progressing. For instance, what if your son were quite ill and you were instructed to take him to the emergency department for observation, but before he left the office he was given his routine vaccines? If he developed a fever while in the emergency department, no one would know if the fever were due to the vaccines or the illness.

## A WEAKENED IMMUNE SYSTEM

Live vaccines (such as measles, mumps, rubella, and chickenpox) should not be given to most children who have weakened immune systems. Their systems may not be able to fight off even the weakened live viruses in the vaccine.

What weakens the immune system?

✛ Any kind of cancer (such as leukemia, lymphoma, sarcoma, brain tumors)

✛ Medicines or radiation to fight cancer. Vaccines usually may be given when the cancer is in remission and the cancer treatments have been discontinued for at least three months.

✛ Inborn immune system weakness (congenital immunodeficiency)

✛ Full-blown AIDS. But persons with HIV infection who don't have symptoms of AIDS may take measles, mumps, rubella, and chickenpox vaccines.

✛ Steroids. But steroids that are given as inhalers or rubbed on the skin are not a problem with live vaccines. Nor are steroids a problem if they are given for fewer than 14 days or only on an every-other-day basis. Low-dose steroids—less than 2 mg for every kilogram of an infant's body weight—do not preclude vaccination.

If someone else in the house has a weakened immune system, your child still can receive live vaccines (except OPV, the live polio vaccine).

## RECEIPT OF BLOOD PRODUCTS

Live vaccines that are injected (such as measles, mumps, rubella, and chickenpox) should not be given to people who have recently received blood transfusions or blood products that have antibodies in them such as immune globulins. The antibodies in the new blood may inactivate the vaccine viruses. You or your healthcare provider can contact the CDC (at 800-232-2522) to request a list that shows how soon a person can receive live injected vaccines after receiving various blood products.

## PREGNANCY

### Vaccines that pregnant women should and should not receive

Live vaccines (such as measles, mumps, rubella, chickenpox) should not be given to pregnant women because, at least in theory, the live vaccine viruses may harm the fetus.

Other vaccines can and should be given. In some countries, all pregnant women are given tetanus vaccine so they will pass protective tetanus antibodies to their offspring. Pregnant women who are at high risk for catching hepatitis B should get that vaccine. Women who are in the last six months of pregnancy during flu season should get flu vaccine to protect themselves. (See the specific disease chapters for details.)

### Pregnancy and vaccinating others in the family

If a mother is pregnant, her children can still safely receive all routinely recommended vaccines. Questions usually arise around the use of live vaccines: measles, mumps, rubella, and chickenpox. Measles, mumps, and rubella vaccine viruses do not spread, so these are of no concern.

Chickenpox vaccine virus cannot spread to someone who is already immune to chickenpox, and almost everyone is immune to chickenpox by the time he or she is an adult. If a pregnant woman believes she never had the disease or the vaccine, then she may be susceptible. The risk of a vaccinated child spreading chickenpox vaccine virus to a susceptible person is quite low, whereas the risk of an unvaccinated child bringing home wild chickenpox virus is still quite high. For this reason, chickenpox vaccine is recommended for routine use even in a household with a pregnant woman who never had the disease.

The live, oral polio vaccine (OPV) is rarely available anymore. If it must be used, then it is acceptable despite the presence of a pregnant woman in the home, but it cannot be used if anyone in the household is not fully vaccinated against polio or has a weakened immune system.

## WHAT OTHER QUESTIONS DO PARENTS ASK?

*Q: Should premature infants be given vaccines later in life than full-term infants?*

Infants who are born prematurely should be vaccinated on the same schedule as full-term infants, with one exception. If the mother is not infected with hepatitis B virus, the baby should weigh 2 kilograms (about 4.5 pounds) before receiving the first hepatitis B vaccine. If the mother is infected with hepatitis B virus, the baby should receive the vaccine within the first 12 hours of life *irrespective of weight*. (See Chapter 8.)

*Q: Does breastfeeding interfere with vaccination?*

If you are breastfeeding, you may take any vaccine without danger to your baby. Similarly, your breast milk will not inactivate the vaccines that your child is given. Rubella vaccine virus (in MMR) has been shown to be in the breast milk of women after taking MMR, but rubella is not transmitted by mouth, so there is no danger to the infant. Breastfeeding women may take MMR and all other necessary vaccines without fear.

*Q: Should we look at family history (such as genes that govern auto-immunity) to see if a child may be at greater risk for problems after vaccination?*

It would be helpful if we could do genetic or any other testing to know who would have a serious reaction, like a life-threatening allergy, after vaccination. But no such test exists.

*Honest differences of views and honest debate are not disunity.*
*They are the vital process of policy-making among free men.*

—Herbert Hoover

Chapter 7

# PARENTS' RIGHTS

The success of the nation's immunization program, ironically, has also become its liability. Since so few wild viruses are still circulating, vaccine side effects receive more attention than the diseases they prevent. "A generation ago," writes a *Newsweek* columnist, "parents...didn't think much about the adverse effects of vaccines"; rather, "they worried about the horrors of infectious disease."

The concern about vaccine side effects comes at the same time as an increase in desire for personal control. "We stand now on the brink of a fundamental shift of power...from institutions more generally to individuals," according to Yankelovich Monitor, a national trends research firm, which interviewed 2,500 consumers aged 16 and older. According to their 1998 report, 95 percent said they "feel it's important to be in control," and 85 percent went so far as to say "It's important to me to feel in charge of each and every part of my life," up from 79 percent in 1995. The researchers also found that many people had less confidence in their healthcare providers than in years past. While in 1988, 71 percent had "a great deal of confidence in advice from doctors," that number had dropped to 58 percent by 1998.

## YOUR OPTIONS

Vanessa Wright, a young mother, states, "I want to be a partner with my child's doctor." But ultimately, Wright says, the right to decide whether her child will receive vaccines should be hers. "I educated myself and considered all the options. I want a doctor who will discuss those options with me and allow me to make the final decision."

Exactly what rights and options do parents have in vaccination decisions that affect their children?

### What is your right to information?

According to the National Childhood Vaccine Injury Act (section 2126 of the U.S. Public Health Service Act) all healthcare providers, *prior* to giving each routinely recommended childhood vaccine, are to provide the parent with a copy of the Vaccine Information Statement (VIS) put out by the CDC and discuss it (see Chapter 2). These sheets tell you about a particular vaccine—what it is, who should and should not receive it, what the risks are, what to do about a moderate or severe reaction, and how to learn more. Though you are supposed to be given this information *before* your child is immunized, you may not receive it unless you ask. It is your right— but also your responsibility—to ask for the information and get the answers to your questions.

### What is your right to report a vaccine side effect?

You have the right to report a vaccine side effect to the Vaccine Adverse Event Reporting System (VAERS). The CDC and the FDA began VAERS in 1990. Healthcare professionals, as well as patients, their families, and manufacturers can report to VAERS any condition they suspect may have been caused by a vaccine. This system accepts and follows up on reports even if there was no medical evaluation of the condition and regardless of when the problem occurred. Since this reporting system is totally voluntary and cases are not confirmed, data may not accurately reflect vaccine safety. The VAERS phone number is 800-822-7967; see the reporting form in Chapter 4 (Figure 4-2).

### What is your right to compensation from a vaccine injury?

The National Vaccine Injury Compensation Program (NVICP) is a federal no-fault system designed to compensate individuals or families thought to have been injured by routine childhood vaccines. You have the right to seek compensation for vaccine injury via this program. The injury or condition must be severe enough to last at least six months. But there is legislation pending that would make it possible for more families to collect damages. Claims are filed through the U.S. Court of Federal Claims, which decides who is eligible for compensation and how much they'll be awarded. So far more than a billion dollars have been paid out to more than 1,400 families since the program began in October 1988. The NVICP phone number is 800-338-2382; the web site address is www.hrsa.gov/bhpr/vicp.

### What are your rights before your child's entry to daycare or school?

You have some options if you are deeply concerned about certain vaccines. Since state immunization laws only require that a child be vaccinated before entering school or, in some states, daycare, you might choose to delay vaccination until you are comfortable that you are doing the right thing for your child. Of course, you should be aware that your child risks getting sick from the given diseases during the wait.

After Cynthia Good's son, Julien, received his DTP shot, he screamed and cried for two hours. Though that alone is not considered a medical contraindication to vaccination, she chose not to let him receive a subsequent dose of the vaccine, knowing the new and improved DTaP vaccine—which promised fewer side effects—soon would be licensed for infants. Just a few months later, DTaP came out and Julien tolerated subsequent doses of it just fine. While it was legal to wait for the vaccine since school entry requirements didn't apply yet, she risked the chance that Julien would get a potentially serious disease.

The personal risks that come with *not* vaccinating are clear. If a highly contagious disease exists in your community and your child is not protected, then he or she may become sick from it. Data collected on children ages 5 to 19 showed that those who were not vaccinated against measles were 35 times more likely to contract the disease than those persons who had received the vaccine. Deciding not to immunize can be dangerous if there is disease in your community, if you are traveling, or even if you are attending a public event. Some vaccine-preventable diseases are so contagious that you can contract the disease from an infected person hundreds of yards away. That's just what happened in the Minneapolis–St. Paul area in 1991 when measles virus was transported through air ducts from one part of a sports arena to another. Because unvaccinated children remain vulnerable, the CDC suggests that parents "consider isolating them (when) a vaccine-preventable disease is known to be causing illness in the community."

## What is your right to a school protected by vaccines?

According to Edward Meivach and colleagues, when parents were presented with the statement, "Parents should be allowed to send their child to school even if not immunized," almost 80 percent of the parents disagreed and almost 66 percent disagreed strongly. The laws that prevent parents from sending their unvaccinated children to school are not federal; state legislatures and even some cities write their own vaccination laws. All schools, public and private, even daycare centers, are required to obtain proof of vaccination or a legal reason for exemption before children are admitted. If an individual is found to be noncompliant, the school must enforce state law by excluding that child from class.

Each state's department of education has responsibility for enforcing the requirements. There is no such thing as the "vaccine police," but if a disease outbreak occurs or a teacher or parent complains, then a noncompliant school could lose its license and government funding. In some states the school principal can even be taken to court, tried, and then fined if found to be operating in violation of state school entry requirements. Of course, some schools and their nurses are stricter than others about making allowances, and only about half of the states have penalty clauses for noncompliance.

State laws requiring immunization date back to 1809 when Massachusetts enacted the smallpox vaccination requirement for its residents. The U.S. Supreme Court has upheld the constitutionality of state school entry vaccination laws twice since then. The first time was in the case *Jacobson v. Massachusetts* in 1905. Jacobson challenged the constitutionality of school immunization laws on grounds that requiring him to be vaccinated constituted an unreasonable infringement of his personal liberty, but the Supreme Court unanimously rejected his argument. The high court ruled that not a single nonimmunized individual should be allowed to enjoy the general protection of an immunized community. Nor would it allow the safety of an entire community to be jeopardized by a single nonimmunized individual who chose to remain a part of that population. The U.S. Supreme Court upheld school immunization laws again in 1922.

## EXEMPTIONS

### What is your right to refuse vaccination?

Some parents have opted to home-school their children rather than to comply with immunization certificate requirements. While those attending public and private schools comply with state-mandated school entry requirements, some private schools have been specifically created for parents who choose not to vaccinate. Still, students at these schools must show valid exemptions.

The types of exemptions offered vary by state and can change with new legislation. Check with your state health department or local school district to see which vaccines are required and which exemptions are permitted this year in your area. Also discuss the rules regarding outbreaks. If an outbreak of a vaccine-preventable disease were to occur in a community, then unvaccinated children should be excluded from school.

**Medical exemptions.** Since January 1998, all states have allowed medical exemptions from school entry vaccination requirements. Physicians are permitted to write medical exemptions for children who are, for example, immuno-compromised or allergic to particular vaccines. To use this exemption a parent or guardian must produce documentation from a licensed physician or from a local board of health prior to the child's entry to school.

**Religious exemptions.** Every state allows religious exemptions, except for Mississippi and West Virginia, where the issue has never been taken to court. The 48 states that do allow religious exemptions have various stipulations. Some require persons requesting an exemption to belong to a church with a written tenet opposing all immunizations. Other states require that a church's spiritual advisor attest to the person's sincere religious objection to vaccination. California, Georgia, and others require only an affidavit stating that the family's religious affiliation opposes vaccination.

The language of religious exemption criteria has been successfully challenged in some states as discriminatory. The Massachusetts Supreme Court held that laws granting exemptions to religious groups that oppose vaccine must also apply to individuals with the same beliefs whether or not they are members of a church.

**Philosophical exemptions.** Fifteen states offer philosophical exemptions. They are Arizona (in elementary and middle school), California, Colorado, Idaho, Louisiana, Maine, Michigan, Minnesota, New Mexico, Ohio, Oklahoma, Utah, Vermont, Washington, and Wisconsin. Nebraska and Missouri offer philosophical exemptions for children in daycare; Missouri also offers them for children in Head Start programs.

The conditions required for philosophical exemption vary from state to state. Usually, parents seeking exemption must sign a document or write a note indicating they are philosophically opposed to childhood immunization. Some states require such a note each year, whereas other states offer a one-time waiver on the school district vaccine record sheet included with registration materials.

## What about community versus individual rights?

The decision not to vaccinate can result in more than your child being kept out of school or even becoming ill. The decision not to vaccinate can result in the introduction of disease into your community.

Clearly when vaccination levels drop, disease incidence and deaths go up. A recent example is the U.S. measles epidemic between 1989 and 1991, which killed 123 people, most commonly in urban areas where immunization levels were low. Similarly, in Great Britain following negative publicity about adverse effects of pertussis vaccine, a drop in pertussis immunizations starting in 1974 was followed in 1978 by an epidemic of more than 100,000 cases and 36 deaths. In Japan in 1974, pertussis immunization levels of 70 percent were accompanied by 393 cases and 0 pertussis-related deaths, but by 1979, with immunization levels down to just 20 to 40 percent, 13,000 pertussis cases and 41 deaths were reported.

It is especially unsafe not to be vaccinated if those around you also are not vaccinated. This has been demonstrated by outbreaks of pertussis, measles, congenital rubella syndrome, and poliomyelitis in unvaccinated religious communities at a time when such diseases were rarely seen in vaccinated Americans. Unvaccinated individuals in communities with a large percentage of unvaccinated people don't benefit from herd immunity. That is, when almost all members of a community (or herd) are vaccinated, then those who are not vaccinated are protected from that disease by the herd. When many members of a community are not vaccinated, the disease circulates freely through the community.

Some children must depend on herd immunity. The vaccines are not 100 percent effective, so a small proportion of vaccinated children remain susceptible. Some children cannot take a particular vaccine because of an allergic reaction to it. Some people with serious health problems, such as compromised immune systems due to cancer, cannot be vaccinated and are at particular danger if infected. These children depend, through no choice of their own, on their community to protect them from disease through herd immunity.

The balance between personal rights and the public good is a fragile one. Members of communities do many things for the good of all, such as not smoking in public places. Clearly, if many of us chose to avoid vaccinations, there would be much more disease around and children who were susceptible—whether by choice or not—would be at much higher risk of getting sick.

## CONCLUSION

Undoubtedly, debate over mandatory vaccination for school will continue. While many public health officials believe that more vaccines should be required if they can reduce disease and death, some antivaccine groups believe that no vaccines should be required at all. In Britain, some parents even hold disease parties; when a child comes down with measles the parents call their friends so other susceptible children can be infected and gain immunity without receiving a shot. That's one way to get around vaccine requirements, though a potentially dangerous one.

Whether you want a vaccine-protected school environment for your child or unrestricted philosophical exemptions, you have the right to contact your congressional representative or legislator and express your opinions, and the right to attend state health department meetings. It's your government, your community, and your child. Make sure your voice gets heard. That way you can affect the future of immunization law.

# PART TWO

---

## Routine Vaccines for Children

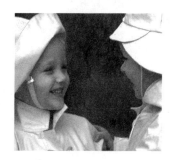

# Chapter 8

# Hepatitis B Vaccine

**Every year in the United States** an estimated 250,000 persons, 35,000 of whom are children, become infected with the hepatitis B virus. About 5,000 die from it. Worldwide, 350 million people are chronically infected, causing 1 to 2 million deaths each year. (See Figure 8-1.)

Hepatitis B vaccine was recommended for all infants in 1991 in the United States, and within five years it was already making an impact. Hepatitis B cases among children ages 3 to 6 declined 62 percent from 1991 to 1996. Among children ages 7 to 10, hepatitis B cases declined by 27 percent. But the full impact of vaccine usage won't be seen until the 2010s and '20s, when children vaccinated today are protected adolescents and adults.

Questions have been raised about whether the vaccine is safe, whether everyone should receive the vaccine even though a U.S.-born child has only a 5 percent risk of infection over a lifetime, and whether the vaccine should routinely be given during infancy when the high-risk period for infection is adulthood. We will answer these and other questions in the sections that follow.

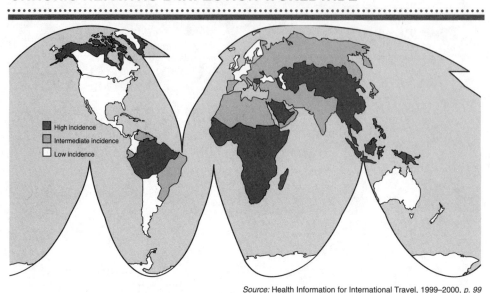

**Figure 8-1**
## CHRONIC HEPATITIS B INFECTION WORLDWIDE

- High incidence
- Intermediate incidence
- Low incidence

*Source:* Health Information for International Travel, 1999–2000, *p. 99*

## THE HEPATITIS B DISEASE

### What is hepatitis B, and how is it spread?

*Hepatitis* means "inflammation of the liver." There is no cure for hepatitis B. Persons who contract the disease either get well, die quickly from an acute infection, or suffer from a long-term, chronic infection. One to 2 percent of infected individuals become severely ill, and 200 Americans die each year from an acute infection. Those persons who become chronically infected die after 20 to 40 years of hepatitis B virus damage to the liver, in the form of liver cirrhosis or liver cancer. Hepatitis B is the most common cause of liver cancer and is second only to smoking as a known cause of cancer.

The virus enters the liver and replicates there, causing symptoms within six weeks to six months. Patients experience nausea, lose their appetite, and show dark urine and jaundice (a yellowing of the skin and the whites of the eyes). Sometimes rashes and joint inflammation are also present.

The younger that persons are when first infected, the less likely they are to develop symptoms soon after infection, but the more likely they are to develop chronic infection. That is, when infected by hepatitis B virus, few infants, 5 to 15 percent of preschool children, and 33 to 50 percent of persons older than 5 develop *symptoms*. But 90 percent of newborns, 25 to 50 percent of preschool children, and 6 to 10 percent of persons older than 5 develop *chronic infection* with all its risks.

Hepatitis B spreads from one human to another by passing into the bloodstream through a break in the skin or the linings of the body cavities (mouth, vagina, or anus). It spreads easily, being 100 times more contagious than HIV, the virus that causes AIDS. Infected persons have large quantities of the hepatitis B virus in their blood, but the virus is also present in lower concentrations in body fluids such as saliva, vaginal fluid, and semen.

Hepatitis B virus may pass through the skin on a contaminated needle during illicit drug use or an improperly performed medical procedure. It may pass through body cavity linings during birth from a mother who is infected.

In some countries, 60 percent of the populace become infected with hepatitis B at some time in their lives, usually during birth or early childhood. As mentioned earlier, Americans have a 5 percent average lifetime risk of becoming infected, usually during adulthood. (See Figure 8-2.)

The groups at greatest risk for infection include heterosexuals who have more than one partner, homosexuals, and injection drug users. Also at risk are people who live with someone who has hepatitis B and healthcare workers who handle blood or needles. About 25 to 30 percent of the people with hepatitis B infection do not report having any risk factor. (See Figure 8-3.)

---

## IT HAPPENED TO A U.S. CONGRESSMAN

United States Congressman John Joseph Moakley hopes all parents will vaccinate their children for hepatitis B. Few know more about the agony the hepatitis B virus can inflict than this congressman from Massachusetts who fought his own battle with it.

Moakley became gravely ill with hepatitis B. The disease led to cirrhosis of the liver and threatened his life. As he waited for a liver transplant, doctors gave him grim news. His scariest moment, he says, was when they "told me I had two months to live." Severely jaundiced, with no strength, he finally received the liver transplant that saved his life. He continues, "After going through that near-death experience, I would stress to anyone the importance of the shot."

Diagnosed in the early 1980s, the congressman still doesn't know how he got hepatitis. He thinks he might have contracted the disease during a congressional fact-finding mission to China. Since he doesn't fit any of the typical risk groups, he explains, "I was surprised. I said, what is hepatitis B? Until that day I was ignorant of hepatitis B. When I, not in a high-risk category, can get it, anyone can. Hepatitis is highly contagious. It doesn't die in the air like HIV."

Congressman Moakley knows that the horror he endured could have been prevented by a simple vaccine.

## Who dies of chronic hepatitis B?

Just as people are more likely to *develop* chronic hepatitis B if they are infected when young, people also are more likely to *die* from complications of chronic hepatitis B if they are infected when young. Among infants and

**Figure 8-2**
## AGE OF ACQUISITION OF HEPATITIS B VIRUS INFECTIONS

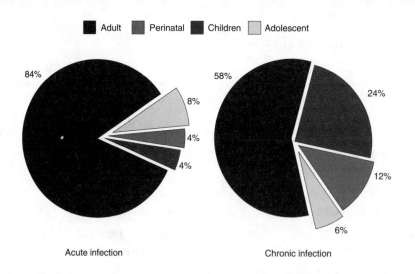

Acute infection

Chronic infection

*Source:* Epidemiology and Prevention, *p. 230*

children who develop a chronic condition, 25 percent will die of cirrhosis or liver cancer. Among adolescents and young adults who acquire a chronic infection, 15 percent will die of hepatitis B. Because hepatitis B usually takes 20 to 40 years to kill a person, most deaths occur in adulthood.

## THE HEPATITIS B VACCINE

### What is hepatitis B vaccine, and how effective is it?

The hepatitis B vaccine is composed of a protein found in the outer envelope of the hepatitis B virus. In the early 1980s, this protein was obtained from the plasma (liquid part of blood) of persons with chronic hepatitis B infection. But fear that other viruses would also be in the blood of persons with chronic hepatitis B prompted development of a safer alternative. Now the protein is produced in yeast cells, not taken from a person's blood. This newer vaccine was licensed in the U.S. in 1986. The original plasma-derived formulation of the vaccine is no longer available in the U.S.

Three doses are recommended in the first year of life. The first dose is generally recommended at birth to 2 months, as long as the infant weighs at least 2 kilograms. If the child's mother has hepatitis B, however, the vaccine should be given to the infant in the first 12 hours of life. (Infants who weigh less than 2 kilograms but whose mothers are infected are at very high risk, so they still should receive the vaccine at birth and then at 1 to 2 months, 4 months, and 6 months of age.)

People who did not receive the vaccine during infancy may receive the vaccine at any age. The ACIP and AAP consider it prudent to give the vaccine by 11 to 12 years of age, if not earlier, so that all three doses are completed well before sexual contact.

**Figure 8-3**

## HEPATITIS B RISK FACTORS

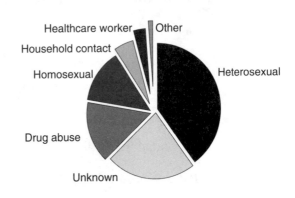

*Source:* Epidemiology and Prevention, *p. 230*

Among children and adults who have not been exposed to the hepatitis B virus, three doses of vaccine protect 95 percent or more of the recipients. Adults age 40 and older do not respond as well to the vaccine.

For persons with normal immune systems, no boosters are recommended because the virus is slow acting. The body has weeks to months to develop a powerful immune response based on its memory of the vaccine. Protection has remained excellent over the almost two decades for which data are available.

## Who should get hepatitis B vaccine and when?

ACIP recommends hepatitis B vaccine for persons who have been exposed to the virus as well as for certain groups prior to exposure. These groups include all children from birth to 19 years of age and all adults at increased risk for infection. Persons at risk include the following:

- ✚ Sexually active heterosexuals who have had more than one sex partner in the previous six months, have a recently acquired sexually transmitted disease, or are being treated for a sexually transmitted disease

- ✚ Men who have sex with men

- ✚ People who live or have sex with someone who has hepatitis B

- ✚ Injection drug users

- ✚ People who, through their occupation, are exposed to blood or blood-contaminated body fluid

- ✚ Clients and staff of institutions for the developmentally disabled

- ✚ Hemodialysis patients and patients with early renal failure

- ✚ Patients who receive clotting-factor concentrates

- ✚ Adoptees from countries where hepatitis B infection is common

- ✚ International travelers who will be in hepatitis B–infected areas for more than 6 months, will have close or sexual contact with residents of those regions, or will have contact with blood (as in a medical setting)

✥ People who will be inmates in a correctional facility for at least four weeks (enough time for two doses of vaccine)

## Who should *not* get the vaccine?

This vaccine should *not* be given to anyone who had a serious allergic reaction to a prior dose of hepatitis B vaccine or its contents (such as baker's yeast). Anyone who has a moderate to severe illness should wait until feeling better to receive the vaccine.

## What are the vaccine risks and side effects?

The most commonly reported side effects are pain and fever. Pain at the injection site is reported by 3 to 29 percent of vaccine recipients, and 1 to 6 percent report temperature greater than 100.9 degrees Fahrenheit. This isn't different from the percentages of such side effects among people who are injected with plain saltwater as a means of comparison. Severe allergic reactions have been reported, but they are rare (roughly 1 in every 600,000 doses). In these rare cases an allergic reaction may range from hives to difficulty breathing, to low blood pressure, to anaphylactic shock.

### IT HAPPENED TO ALEXANDRA

Alexandra had an adverse reaction to the hepatitis B vaccine. Dan Burton, a U.S. congressman from Indiana, says his first grandchild, a healthy baby girl, had no problem with her initial hepatitis B vaccine at birth. But, he says, following her second dose of the vaccine, when she was a month old, little Alexandra "screamed constantly" and "developed a fever." That night in December 1993, ten minutes after she had been put to bed, her parents checked on her and found that she had stopped breathing. "They rushed her to the hospital," he recalls. "She threw up and went into a convulsion." She was in the hospital for two weeks. "We thought she was going to die." For six months, little Alexandra remained on an apnea monitor to make sure she continued to breathe.

Today Alexandra is a healthy, bright, and energetic 6 year old. Still, her grandfather is angry that his daughter, Alexandra's mother, had not been told that a severe reaction to the vaccine was even a possibility. Congressman Burton says, "It's important the parent has a clear understanding of the possible side effects, and I think parents ought to have the right to defer action on the vaccine until later." He adds, "I believe vaccinations are important," but parents need to be fully informed about side effects "so they can participate in the decision-making process."

In fact, it is every parent's right to receive, prior to the child's immunization, a Vaccine Information Statement, which states potential adverse reactions. Serious allergic reactions are rare following hepatitis B vaccine.

## Other vaccine safety concerns

In the United States more than 20 million adults and adolescents and more than 16 million infants and children have received hepatitis B vaccine; worldwide, more than 500 million people have received the vaccine. Because very few serious side effects have been noted after millions of doses, the World Health Organization, the CDC, the American Academy of Pediatrics, and the American Academy of Family Physicians all consider the vaccine quite safe.

Two major scientific summaries have been published on hepatitis B vaccine risks.

1. The U.S. Food and Drug Administration reviewed reports found in the Vaccine Adverse Event Reporting System (VAERS) from 1991 to 1994 and found no unexpected adverse events in neonates and infants given hepatitis B vaccine, despite the use of at least 12 million doses of vaccine in these age groups.

2. Grotto and colleagues reviewed the world's medical literature and found that hepatitis B vaccine reactions were rare, but that the reported reactions were similar to those occurring after hepatitis B disease.

**Multiple sclerosis (MS).** MS is a disease that causes myelin nerve covers to degenerate, thereby causing marked muscle weakness. It is most common in young adult females, especially those in northern latitudes. Case reports of individuals who developed MS within two to three months after hepatitis B vaccination have suggested an association between these two. Between 1990 and the summer of 1999, 76 such cases were reported to the VAERS. Although MS often develops during young adulthood, the same age that people frequently receive hepatitis B vaccine, the similarity in time frame does not mean that one causes the other.

Two expert panels have reviewed the data and have found no scientific evidence of a relationship between hepatitis B vaccine and MS or other demyelinating disorders. In 1998, the National Multiple Sclerosis Society reported "no current evidence of a link between hepatitis B vaccination and MS." The European Viral Hepatitis Prevention Board of the World Health Organization and the French government had come to the same conclusion in 1997. Additional studies are being conducted.

**Guillain-Barré syndrome.** When the VAERS indicated a possible link between this paralyzing disease of the nerves and hepatitis B vaccine, the CDC and the FDA analyzed the data. They found that GBS was no more frequent among vaccinated than among unvaccinated people.

**Hair loss.** More than 45 people have reported hair loss after receiving this vaccine; less than a third of these had permanent hair loss. However, a study of a large number of people in a managed care organization showed that having received hepatitis B vaccine did not influence a person's chance of hair loss.

**Sudden Infant Death syndrome.** SIDS, or crib death, has been reported after hepatitis B vaccination. However, the incidence of reported SIDS deaths was higher before hepatitis B vaccine was widely used. Specifically, in 1992, only 8 percent (320,000) of U.S. infants received the vaccine, and 4,800 SIDS deaths were reported. In 1996, when the number of infants in the U.S. was roughly the same as it was in 1992, 82 percent of U.S. infants received the vaccine, and only 3,000 SIDS deaths were reported. SIDS deaths are even less frequent now. The drop in SIDS deaths at a time when millions more infants are being vaccinated indicates that hepatitis B vaccine is probably not a cause of SIDS.

## WHAT OTHER QUESTIONS DO PARENTS ASK?

*Q: Why give the vaccine to newborn babies when the disease only affects adults and when newborns are at lower risk?*

Originally, the U.S. plan for preventing hepatitis B was to give the vaccine to adults who were at risk for the disease. It was a logical, focused approach. Unfortunately, it did not work, in part because adults usually don't seek healthcare unless they are already ill. Another reason the strategy did not work is because hepatitis B virus is not limited to adults. Though only a small *percentage* of the children in the U.S. become infected each year with hepatitis B, the *number* of children is as high as 35,000. Also, the children who are infected are more likely to have chronic infection and to die from that infection.

*Q: I don't think my child will ever be in an at-risk group (such as IV drug users, highly sexually active heterosexuals, or homosexuals), so why should he receive the vaccine?*

Persons who are not in a high-risk group still need the vaccine because up to 30 percent of individuals infected with hepatitis B virus (as many as 90,000 persons each year) had no known risk factor for infection.

*Q: When will we see proof that the strategy to immunize babies works?*

In the U.S. the hepatitis B vaccine is already having a positive impact. According to Eric Mast of the CDC, between 1991 and 1996, rates of acute hepatitis B declined by 62 percent in children ages 3 to 6 and declined 27 percent in children ages 7 to 10.

Studies show that the use of the vaccine has already decreased the incidence of hepatitis B virus in children in China, Gambia, and American Samoa. Liver cancer has decreased among vaccinated children in Taiwan where the vaccine is routinely administered to infants.

*Q: If the mother is tested for hepatitis B and she is not infected, does the infant still need the vaccine?*

Being born to a hepatitis B–infected mother puts a child at risk, but many children are infected in other ways. A study in 1990 estimated that among children less than 10 years of age born in the U.S. to mothers who were not hepatitis B infected, more than 33,000 were infected by hepatitis B virus. This translates to a risk of approximately 85 per 100,000.

*Q: Isn't it enough to counsel adolescents about hepatitis B risk factors (such as sexual activity, exposure to blood products, and intravenous drug use) rather than vaccinate?*

When the hepatitis B vaccine first was licensed in the U.S. this strategy was used, but it was not effective. Usually, adolescents and adults don't seek healthcare unless they are ill, so there is little opportunity for counseling. By the time someone is identified as being in a high-risk group, he or she may already be infected. It is important that people receive three doses of the vaccine before they are exposed to the virus.

*Q: How do hepatitis A, hepatitis B, and hepatitis C differ from each other?*

The viruses that cause hepatitis A, B, and C are not even related to each other, so they behave quite differently. For example, hepatitis A is spread in stool, whereas the other two are spread in blood and body fluids. Despite these differences, it would be hard to tell them apart just from the symptoms they cause.

*Q: Is it true that the French no longer use hepatitis B vaccine?*

No, the French still use this vaccine, but in October 1998 the French Ministry of Health announced the decision to discontinue their school-based hepatitis B immunization program for adolescents. It was felt that, because parents were not present in schools to discuss the risks and benefits of vaccination, it would be better if adolescents were encouraged to receive the vaccine during doctor visits—as infants do.

## WHAT DOES THE FUTURE HOLD?

An advisory group to the World Health Organization has recommended that all countries include hepatitis B vaccine in their national immunization programs. One hundred countries have already done so. Often the poorest countries have been unable make hepatitis B available because the vaccine is relatively expensive.

In Taiwan, liver cancer deaths have dropped dramatically since the start of the hepatitis B vaccination program in the 1980s. In the U.S., ongoing data collection will be necessary to show that the hepatitis B vaccine is completely safe, that its protection is lasting, and that the current strategy is worth its cost.

*Humanity has but three great enemies: fever, famine, and war; of these, by far the greatest, by far the most terrible, is fever.*

—Sir William Osler

Chapter 9

# DTaP Vaccine:
## Diphtheria, Tetanus, and Acellular Pertussis

Diphtheria, tetanus, and pertussis (or whooping cough) are prevented by one combined vaccine, DTaP. Each of the three diseases was a major killer, so use of the combined vaccine became routine practice in the 1940s.

DTP, the early version of the present vaccine, often caused frightening side effects in infants and children, which in turn prompted vocal and organized opposition to the vaccine in this and other developed countries. In large part, DTP's problem was that the pertussis component was produced by killing pertussis bacteria cells and then using the whole, killed cell in the vaccine. The whole-cell vaccine contained not only the parts of the bacteria that induced immunity, but also parts that caused fever and other side effects. For more than twenty years, scientists worked to identify and purify the exact parts of the cell that would induce immunity but not cause severe side effects. In 1981, a safer pertussis vaccine was licensed in Japan that did not contain whole cells; it was *acellular.*

Ten years later, in 1991, the first acellular pertussis vaccine was licensed for booster doses in the U.S. In 1996, DTaP was also licensed for the infant doses. By 1999, the acellular pertussis vaccine had been so widely accepted that ACIP and the American Academy of Pediatrics expressed their preference for this formulation by including only DTaP in the routine childhood immunization schedule. The marked decrease in demand for the older DTP is leading to its withdrawal from the U.S. market.

## DIPHTHERIA

From 1860 to 1897 in Massachusetts (one of the only states that kept public health statistics then), 3 to 10 percent of *all* deaths were caused by diphtheria. In the United States by the 1920s, the disease was reported in 100,000 to 200,000 people each year (many cases were not reported), and it killed 13,000 to 15,000 of them. Once the vaccine became available in the late 1940s, the number of persons infected with the disease began to drop. By the 1980s, on average only three cases were reported each year, and diphtheria deaths became a thing of the past.

Though the vaccine has been available for more than half a century, countries still need to make sure that children are vaccinated and that adults receive boosters. Diphtheria outbreaks have occurred recently in eastern Europe, Russia, Brazil, Nigeria, India, Indonesia, and the Philippines. In eastern Europe and Russia in particular, decreased immunization rates and lack of an adult vaccination program are blamed for an increase in cases.

### What is diphtheria, and how is it spread?

Humans are not the only ones infected by viruses. In diphtheria, the bacteria *Corynebacterium diphtheriae* become infected by a virus and start producing a poison. If, for example, a person's throat is infected with the poison-producing bacteria, then the poison penetrates the surrounding cells and kills them. Debris from dying cells and inflammation gradually form a membrane that adheres closely to the lining of the throat at first, but then sloughs. When it sloughs, it can block the airway. (See Figure 9-1)

As if this were not enough, the poison that gets into the bloodstream can damage tissues elsewhere in the person's body. The heart, the kidneys, and the nervous system are prime targets. Inflammation and tissue destruction in these organs cause diphtheria's complications. The nerves that serve muscles may be temporarily inflamed, and if the breathing muscles are involved, then the disease can lead to pneumonia and respiratory failure. Abnormal function of the heart can occur after the first or second week of illness, and it's usually irreversible.

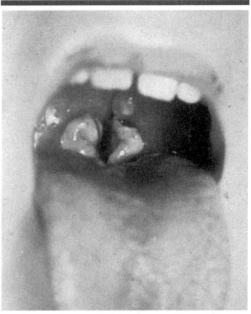

**Figure 9-1**
**DIPHTHERIA (tonsillar)**

Source: CDC

Even in mild cases, the death rate is high unless patients are treated. Overall, 5 to 10 percent of patients who catch diphtheria die from it, even in the modern medical age.

Some humans carry and shed the bacteria without symptoms. These carriers, as well as infected individuals who are ill with diphtheria, spread the disease directly to other people by sneezing, coughing, and speaking. Though the germ is hardy, doctors do not know if it can be passed on a soiled object such as a drinking cup, used facial tissue, or toothbrush.

Since 1980, diphtheria has been reported most frequently in people younger than 10 or older than 50 years old. It is likely that the children were incompletely vaccinated and that the seniors had not had boosters in many years.

### IT HAPPENED IN RUSSIA

In June 1995, the CDC sent Dr. Chuck Vitek to Russia to do research on diphtheria. "The saddest cases were kids who had not been vaccinated and went on to die," he says. He speaks of a 13-year-old girl who developed heart damage, as is common in severe cases of diphtheria. Vitek explains the girl couldn't talk because she had a tube in her trachea so she could breathe; but she did smile at him. Because there was nothing he or any of the other doctors could do once she developed the heart damage, the girl soon died from heart failure.

Vitek says this was especially sad since the girl probably would have been fine had she simply received the vaccine to prevent diphtheria. The girl's parents decided not to immunize her out of fear that side effects from the vaccine might hurt their daughter because she was mildly mentally retarded, Vitek says. What happened to her, he says, was far worse than any side effects, which are uncommon with this vaccine. "It's hard to see a girl die when that death could have been easily prevented," Vitek states.

Vitek saw infectious disease hospitals filled with sick people. During the epidemic, from 1990 to 1998, more than 150,000 people became sick from diphtheria and more than 5,000 people died from the disease in the countries of the former Soviet Union. Vitek blames the epidemic largely on declining vaccination rates due to "parental resistance to vaccine." He says that often when vaccines do their job, people "appreciate them less." Russians associated mandatory vaccination with the excesses of the communist period. When vaccination rates dropped, "the diphtheria bacteria multiplied and spread," Vitek explains. "The epidemic started in big cities and then spread out to the countryside."

Vitek watched victims of diphtheria flow into hospitals. "Most came in with bad sore throats and a high fever. In more severe cases they would have trouble breathing. Some went on to have heart failure."

"Some of those who were immunized did get sick," he notes, "but I didn't see any of them die. It made me appreciate the fact that preventing the disease is a lot easier than fixing it afterward."

"There is still some diphtheria in the United States," he reminds us. And "outside of the continental U.S., there is lots of diphtheria."

## TETANUS

This painful disease, which often results in death, was not uncommon in the United States in the nineteenth century. Wound management improved, and then in 1924 the first tetanus vaccine was produced. Up to that point, as many as 1500 persons contracted tetanus each year. A marked decrease in deaths occurred between the early 1900s and the late 1940s, when 500 to 600 cases were reported each year, causing 180 deaths. After the 1940s, the tetanus rates fell steadily, averaging fewer than 70 cases and 15 deaths per year. An all-time low of 36 cases was reported in 1996.

Tetanus in the newborn period occurs when mothers do not have tetanus antibodies to pass to their fetuses. Often the umbilical stump is infected because of improper cord care. The tetanus death rate in newborns is 95 percent without treatment. In the U.S. in 1900, 64 out of 100,000 infants less than 1 year of age died of tetanus. Since 1989, only two cases of tetanus in newborns have been reported in the U.S., but worldwide 270,000 newborns and 30,000 mothers still die annually.

Unfortunately, because the tetanus spores are ever present in the earth, we will never eradicate the disease. But the availability of the tetanus vaccine enables us to prevent persons from contracting the disease.

## What is tetanus, and how is it spread?

Tetanus spores, which are scattered all over the earth, are so tough that they easily tolerate being sprayed with antiseptics or being heated to 250 degrees Fahrenheit for 10 to 15 minutes. They live in soil and street dust, and even in the bowels and stools of many domestic and farm animals. Tetanus is *not* contagious. One person cannot catch it from another person.

Occasionally a susceptible person gets a puncture wound, a dental or ear infection, or an animal bite, and the wound is contaminated with tetanus spores (see Figure 9-2). In the wound, the spores germinate and begin to produce a poison. The poison blocks the nerve impulses that

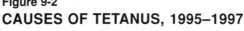

**Figure 9-2**
## CAUSES OF TETANUS, 1995–1997

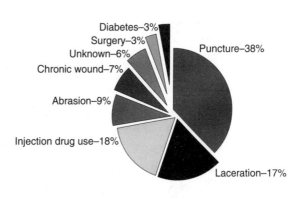

Diabetes–3%
Surgery–3%
Unknown–6%
Chronic wound–7%
Abrasion–9%
Injection drug use–18%
Puncture–38%
Laceration–17%

*Source:* Epidemiology and Prevention, *p. 62*

**Figure 9–3**

**TETANUS (adult; this spasm bends the head and heels back and the hips forward)**

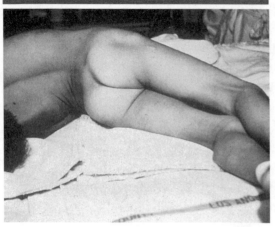

*Source: CDC*

allow muscle relaxation, so the result is excruciating muscle spasms. The muscle spasms are so strong they can crack thighbones and vertebrae. (See Figure 9-3.) The spasms also prevent the essential processes of swallowing and breathing. The most common form of death from tetanus is suffocation, because its victims cannot breathe.

Almost all reported cases of tetanus are in persons who either were never vaccinated or did not receive a booster within the ten years prior to the wound. From 1982 to 1997 in the U.S., two-thirds of the persons who developed tetanus were 50 or older.

## IT HAPPENED TO AN ELDERLY WOMAN

Because of high vaccination coverage levels, few people suffer the devastation of tetanus. It's a good thing. Dr. William Atkinson, an epidemiologist in the National Immunization Program at CDC, offers a sense of the horror that comes with this vaccine-preventable disease.

Dr. Atkinson treated a woman in her late sixties who had injured herself in the garden. She had contracted tetanus, probably from a puncture wound from a thorny bush. She was admitted to the hospital with muscle spasms, then went into respiratory arrest. Doctors had to put her on a ventilator due to the continuous painful spasms.

The woman remained in the intensive care unit for nearly a month. She stayed on a ventilator and on morphine and tranquilizers. She couldn't open her mouth or breathe. "That's the worst suffering I've ever seen," Atkinson says, "and you can't do anything about it."

Later, when asked, the woman couldn't say whether she had ever been immunized against tetanus. The vaccine was not invented until she was a young adult. Without medical intervention she surely would have died from tetanus.

But this story doesn't end happily. No longer paralyzed and on a ventilator, after the disease had run its course, she was moved to a regular hospital room. After being bedridden and sick for so long, she could barely move. She had been in the hospital for six weeks when she developed a blood clot in her leg that moved to her lungs and killed her. She died as a result of being hospitalized for tetanus. Atkinson notes that often if tetanus victims do not die from suffocation, they may die following long periods of immobility and hospitalization.

## PERTUSSIS (WHOOPING COUGH)

In the 1920s, U.S. healthcare providers and labs were first required to report cases of pertussis. For the next twenty years, 115,000 to 270,000 cases resulting in 5,000 to 10,000 deaths were reported each year. The pertussis vaccine became available and began to be widely used in the 1940s; the number of cases then followed a bumpy trend downward. (See Figure 9-4A).

But after 1976, progress stopped. The number of reported cases of pertussis rose from 1,010 in that year to 6,279 in 1998. (See Figure 9-4B.) Reasons suggested for the increase have included use of a vaccine that is not as effective as believed, the natural cycles of the disease, and stepped-up surveillance of the disease (especially among adults).

Time and again, history has shown how persistent pertussis is and how dangerous it is to become lax in vaccinating children against the disease. Following bad press about DTP in 1975, the Japanese government put a moratorium on the vaccine. The number of pertussis cases rose from a few hundred to some 13,000 cases and more than 110 related deaths. Worldwide, in 1944, pertussis caused an estimated 40 million infections that resulted in 5 million cases of pneumonia and 360,000 deaths. Fifty thousand survivors were left with long-term nervous system disorders, including brain damage. Complicating factors like low birth weight and malnutrition, as well as other infections, particularly of the digestive tract or lungs, make pertussis more deadly, so pertussis vaccine is of great importance in developing countries.

## Figure 9-4A
## PERTUSSIS IN THE UNITED STATES, 1940–1998

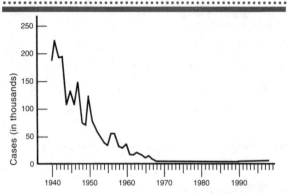

Source: Epidemiology and Prevention, p. 72

## What is pertussis, and how is it spread?

A bacterium called *Bordetella pertussis* causes pertussis (whooping cough). The bacteria produce a poison, which inflames the airway and paralyzes the tiny hairlike fibers, called cilia, that normally sway to move mucus and other debris up the airway, away from the lungs. When cilia are paralyzed, mucus builds up, and the airway becomes blocked. It becomes increasingly difficult to pass air through the inflamed, blocked airway, especially for infants, who have relatively narrow airways. Pneumonia is the most common complication of pertussis (10 percent), followed by seizures (1 percent), inflammation of the brain (0.2 percent), and death (0.2 percent).

In the early stages, pertussis seems like a common cold that won't let go for one or two weeks. Then the young patient develops severe coughing fits, trying to clear the heavy coat of mucus from the airway. After many powerful coughs, the child, trying to breath in, inhales so desperately that the effort creates a high-pitched whoop. Children often vomit after coughing jags and become exhausted. Eating and drinking become difficult if the breaks between coughing spells are insufficient. Finally, after one to six weeks, gradual recovery begins, but for months recovery may be interspersed with relapses when other respiratory infections set in. From 1990 to 1996, about one-third of all persons with pertussis, and almost three-quarters of infants

## Figure 9-4B
## PERTUSSIS IN THE UNITED STATES, 1980–1998

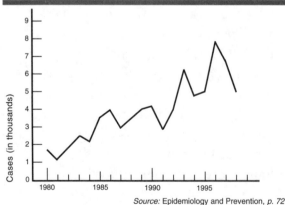

Source: Epidemiology and Prevention, p. 72

less than 6 months old with the disease, needed to be hospitalized. (See Figure 9-5.)

Pertussis is highly contagious. Seventy to 100 percent of those persons who are not immunized against pertussis will contract the disease when exposed. Pertussis is spread by microscopic droplets of mucus coughed or sneezed from an infected person. A vulnerable person might breathe them into the lungs or transfer them to the nose or throat on dirty fingers.

Pertussis is more severe and therefore more frequently reported in infants and children than in adolescents or adults, who usually experience pertussis as a common cold. Some adults develop a prolonged cough and miss a lot of work, but more importantly, early in the course of the disease they spread it to co-workers or classmates, as well as to the children they live with. With increased recognition of the incidence and danger of pertussis in older people, reporting patterns are changing. From 1985 to 1987, 25 percent of reported cases were in persons older than 10 years of age; but from 1995 to 1998, 42 percent of reported cases were in this age group.

**Figure 9-5**
## PERTUSSIS COMPLICATIONS BY AGE, 1990–1996

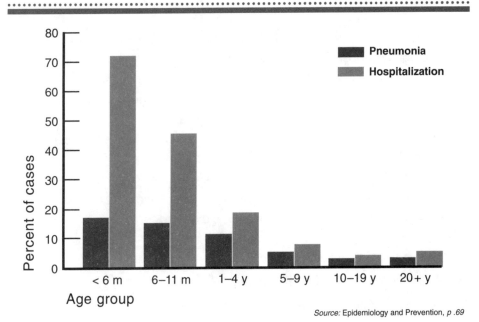

*Source:* Epidemiology and Prevention, *p .69*

## It Happened To Kristal's Twins

"My doctor told me that had I waited one more day to bring my babies in, they would have been dead," said Kristal Weicht, mother of newborn twins.

Kristal took her babies, Klaudia and Justin, to the doctor after they developed coughs. At just 1 month old, Klaudia "started gasping for air," Kristal explains. The doctor said, "give her a steam." It didn't work. So the next day, Kristal took her babies to the emergency room where the pediatrician diagnosed bronchitis. After Kristal took them home with the recommended prescription, Klaudia, clearly the more seriously ill of the two, stopped breathing and turned blue. "She went limp in my arms, and her eyes turned back into her head. I called 911." But by the time paramedics arrived, Klaudia luckily had begun breathing on her own again.

When Kristal took the babies back to the pediatrician, Klaudia stopped breathing again—this time in front of a nurse. Finally the skeptical doctor ordered oxygen and sent both infants to the emergency room. They were admitted to the hospital, where they spent the first two weeks in ICU. They remained hospitalized for two full months. Kristal lived in the hospital room, standing watch over her babies.

Five days into their stay, a nasal culture came back positive for pertussis for both Justin and Klaudia. Kristal says, "they didn't suspect it because it wasn't winter, the typical time of year for pertussis."

Kristal is relieved her babies are recovering. She knows now she acted appropriately, even though "a lot of people told me I was an over-reactive mother." She can't quite shake the sight of her tiny babies dependent on breathing and feeding tubes.

And Kristal is angry. Because of financial reasons, Kristal had to return to work and put her twins in daycare shortly after their birth. She believes her babies, too young to be vaccinated, were exposed to pertussis at daycare.

Kristal says, "I wish babies could get these shots earlier so they would be protected from diseases like pertussis."

"I'm so happy they're okay," she says, holding the babies. "For a while I was scared they wouldn't be. It's the most wonderful thing to know they're going to be okay."

## THE DTaP VACCINE

### What is DTaP vaccine, and how effective is it?

The diphtheria and tetanus portions of the vaccine are made by taking the diseases' poisons and altering them so they're not dangerous anymore. The pertussis vaccine varies from manufacturer to manufacturer, but each contains various parts of the pertussis bacteria.

The vaccine usually is given at 2, 4, and 6 months of age. A booster may be given any time from 12 to 18 months of age and again at 4 to 6 years of age, before the child enters school. The current pertussis vaccines are reported to be from 59 to 89 percent effective, so it's important for young children to receive the full five-dose series.

Tetanus and diphtheria boosters (without pertussis) are given at 11 to 12 years of age and every 10 years thereafter. It's recommended that people get their adult boosters around their twentieth, thirtieth, fortieth birthdays, and so on, so it is easier to remember.

### Who should get DTaP vaccine and when?

All children should get these vaccines. Adolescents and adults should get tetanus-diphtheria boosters, but there is no pertussis vaccine for persons 7 years of age or older. Because the whole-cell pertussis vaccine caused many side effects in adults, and because the disease is not severe in older children and adults, no pertussis vaccine has been licensed for adults. Now that healthcare authorities are learning about the role that these older groups play in spreading the disease, however, an acellular vaccine is in development for them.

### Who should *not* get the vaccine?

If your child had any of the following conditions within 48 to 72 hours of a previous dose of DTP or DTaP, the benefits and risks of more doses must be weighed carefully. You and your physician may decide to give just the diphtheria and tetanus portions of the vaccine and withhold the pertussis part.

✥ Temperature of 105°F or greater without another identifiable cause

✥ Collapse or shocklike state

✥ Persistent crying for three hours or more

✥ A seizure with or without a fever

This vaccine also should not be given to children who

✥ Are younger than 6 weeks or older than 7 years of age.

✥ Had a serious allergic reaction to a prior dose of DTaP, DTP, or any of the vaccine components.

✥ Had encephalopathy, a sudden and severe disorder of the brain, within seven days of a previous dose of a pertussis-containing vaccine. This is a severe condition that manifests as disorientation or even coma, or as seizures that persist for more than a few hours. Encephalopathy requires hospitalization.

✥ Has a moderate to severe illness. If this is the case, the child may receive the vaccine when feeling better.

## What are the vaccine risks and side effects?

Vaccine efficacy trials in Europe for the improved DTaP showed the first three doses of the new acellular pertussis vaccine cut side effects substantially. Forty to 73 percent of persons who received the DTP (old/whole cell vaccine) had local reactions, while only 4 to 40 percent of those who received the DTaP (new/acellular vaccine) had local reactions. Sixteen percent of persons who received the DTP developed a fever over 100 degrees, but only 3 to 5 percent of those who received the DTaP developed a fever over 101 degrees.

More recent data from the Vaccine Adverse Events Reporting System confirm a dramatic reduction in reports of adverse events following DTaP.

Dr. Gina Mootrey at the National Immunization Program compiled VAERS numbers which show a 30 percent overall decrease in side effects following vaccination with DTaP compared to DTP, a 33 percent decrease in mild side effects such as fever and pain at the injection site, and a 25 percent decrease in serious side effects. These data corroborate the findings of the prelicensure clinical trials.

Parents can expect the following reactions to the DTaP vaccine:

✛ Pain or tenderness in 46 out of 1,000 children

✛ Swelling at the site of the injection in 80 out of 1,000 children

✛ Fussiness in 300 out of 1,000 children

✛ Low fever in 58 out of 1,000 children

✛ High fever (over 105°F) in 1 out of 3,000 children

✛ Crying longer than 3 hours in 1 out of 2,000 children

✛ Limpness or paleness in 1 out of 14,300 children

✛ Convulsions or seizures in 1 out of 14,300 children

DTaP is now recommended for all five doses. Now, infants who were started on DTaP can complete their series with DTaP. But Melinda Wharton (Chief of the Child Vaccine Preventable Diseases Branch of the CDC National Immunization Program) points out, in reference to the fourth and fifth doses of DTaP, "As more studies are done, it has become clear that the reactions seen with acellular pertussis vaccines do increase as more doses are given. We're talking about local reactions at the injection site, redness, and swelling mostly, sometimes with pain or sometimes with itching." According to the CDC, "available data suggest a substantial increase in the frequency and magnitude of local reactions with the fourth and fifth doses. Twenty to 30 percent develop erythema or tenderness, and 5 to 10 percent report a temperature of 100 degrees or higher."

As noted above, the whole-cell pertussis vaccine on rare occasions has caused a disorder of the central nervous system called encephalopathy. It consisted of decreased alertness, unresponsiveness, or seizures that persisted more than a few hours. Encephalopathy has not yet been associated with the new acellular vaccine.

## IT HAPPENED TO LAURA

Laura had a serious adverse reaction to the DTP vaccine, according to her mother, Carol Meyer.

Six-week-old Laura, from Wichita, Kansas, received her first DTP vaccine during a well-baby checkup back in 1983. Her mother says that within twelve hours Laura screamed a high-pitched cry. "I'd never heard her cry like that before or after that day." She also says Laura had two brief, mild seizures. But that night, Carol says, Laura suffered a nine-minute generalized seizure. "It affected her whole body." Afterward the infant appeared fine, and the doctor told Carol to bring the baby in the next day. Carol says the doctor told her that very little had been written about this sort of reaction to DTP.

"From that day on," Carol recalls, Laura "was having seizures every other day." Holding back tears, Carol explains that "it got to the point that for the rest of her life we had to watch her every second." At 5 or 6 months of age, Laura began having "status seizures," which lasted up to an hour.

Years later, at age 7, Laura learned to "crawl a little bit," but she remained in diapers and never learned to speak. Still, Carol says, Laura was a happy child. She describes Laura as "beautiful, lovable, easygoing. She would smile. We were really lucky. I never saw her mad, angry, or frustrated."

In 1990, following testimony from a pediatric neurologist and their family doctor, the Meyer family received compensation from the National Vaccine Injury Compensation Program.

Laura passed away at age 11 due to respiratory failure and cardiac arrest. "She was a real gift for us," her mother says. "She taught us so much. We loved her. We thank God for her."

The Meyers' two older children never had a problem following vaccination. Rare reactions, like the one Laura experienced after DTP, led to the DTaP vaccine, which has caused fewer side effects.

## WHAT OTHER QUESTIONS DO PARENTS ASK?

*Q: Does the pertussis vaccine cause SIDS?*

No, quite the opposite. Sudden Infant Death syndrome (SIDS), or crib death, has been associated with DTP largely because the vaccine was used in the first year or life, which is also when crib death occurs. The National Institute of Child Health and Human Development (part of the National Institutes of Health) conducted a large study and found a lowered risk for SIDS in children who had received DTP vaccine.

*Q: Does the vaccine cause autism?*

In January 1990, an Institute of Medicine committee examining possible adverse events associated with DTP vaccine concluded that there was no evidence to indicate a causal relation between DTP vaccine or the pertussis component of DPT vaccine and autism.

*Q: Have some lots of DTaP vaccine been recalled?*

Yes. On January 26, 1999, Pasteur-Merieux Connaught, USA (now called Aventis Pasteur), voluntarily recalled Tripedia DTaP vaccine, lot #0916490, distributed between February and June 1998. Routine testing determined that the potency of the diphtheria component, acceptable at the time of release, had fallen below acceptable specifications.

*Q: Why can't my child receive DTaP earlier so he can be protected sooner?*

The vaccine is not licensed for use before 6 weeks of age. There are not enough data to show it is safe and effective before then.

*Q: Can allergic reactions also occur with this newer acellular vaccine?*

Yes. If a child had a severe allergic reaction to the old DTP or to DTaP, an allergist should be consulted. It is possible that the allergist can determine if, for example, the child can safely take the diphtheria and tetanus vaccine.

*Q: Should I be concerned about the effectiveness of DTP or DTaP wearing off after a while?*

Yes. The vaccine is not expected to be effective for more than 10 years, so boosters of diphtheria and tetanus vaccines are recommended every 10 years. Someday, there may be an adult pertussis booster.

*Q: Is this vaccine worth the risk since a lot of times it doesn't work?*

Almost no one would dispute that the diphtheria and tetanus components of this vaccine are worthwhile, because the risks are minimal and the benefits are great. The pertussis component is the only portion that is controversial. The pertussis vaccine is much less controversial since the new acellular vaccine became available and resulted in a dramatic reduction in side effects. However, parents do need to be aware that the current pertussis vaccines may not be as effective (reports range from 59 to 89 percent) as, for example, measles vaccine (90 to 98 percent). All five shots (the entire three-dose infant series plus the two boosters) are necessary for maximal protection. Of course, when compared to fully vaccinated children, many more who have not received pertussis vaccine will contract whooping cough.

## WHAT DOES THE FUTURE HOLD?

Although most reported cases of pertussis are in children and the severity of the disease is greatest in infancy, the role of adults in spreading pertussis has piqued interest. Vaccinating adults in a household may protect infants too young to have completed their immunizations. Vaccinating adults against pertussis may also decrease their symptoms and consequent absenteeism from work due to severe and persistent cough. At this time, no pertussis vaccine is licensed for adults, but a time may come when it is added to the routine tetanus-diphtheria booster.

*We had all been caught up in the polio epidemic: the early neighbor boy who wore one tall shoe, to which his despairing father added another two soles every year; the girl in the iron lung reading her schoolbook in an elaborate series of mirrors while a volunteer waited to turn the page; my friend who limped, my friend who rolled everywhere in a wheelchair, my friend whose arm hung down, Mother's friend who walked with crutches. My beloved...aunt...had come to visit one day and, while she was saying hello, flung herself on the couch in tears; her son had it.*

—Annie Dillard

# Chapter 10

# Polio Vaccine

Before the polio vaccine was licensed in 1955, polio disease was rampant in the United States and other developed countries. In 1952 alone, polio left more than 20,000 Americans paralyzed. By 1965, the number of Americans paralyzed from polio each year had dropped to 61. Thanks to the vaccine, since 1979 not a single case of natural, or wild, polio has been contracted in the United States. Since 1991, not a single case of wild polio has been contracted in the entire Western Hemisphere.

Polio infection is most common among children, but infected adults are more likely to be paralyzed by the disease. Also, while polio kills 2 to 5 percent of children afflicted by the disease, it kills 15 to 30 percent of affected adults.

Polio has maimed and killed humans through the centuries. Even drawings from ancient Egypt depict humans who appear to have the withered limb of polio. If polio has been around for that long, why did polio epidemics start in Europe in the early 1800s and worsen in developed nations over the next hundred years? One theory is that polio outbreaks occurred because sanitary conditions improved.

Two hundred years ago, nearly all infants were exposed to poliovirus when they still had some of their mother's antibodies in their bloodstreams. Their immunity to poliovirus was boosted as they were exposed over and over, throughout life, so the proportion of people who were paralyzed by the disease was relatively low. As sanitary conditions improved, infants were less likely to be exposed to the virus. Older children and adults being exposed for the first time were more likely to develop paralytic disease.

By the early 1950s, an average of more than 20,000 persons contracted paralytic polio in the United States each year. Parents were terrorized by the fear of polio.

No wild polio has originated in the United States since 1979, but five cases were imported between 1980 and 1989. Outbreaks of polio continue to occur in sub-Saharan Africa, India, and the countries contiguous with India (see Figure 10-1).

Polio has been one of the most scrutinized vaccines for two reasons. First, polio has almost been eradicated from the globe, so many parents ask why the vaccine is needed at all. Although we are close to global eradication, worldwide there were still several thousand cases of polio in 1999, and the virus is easily imported and spread. Until the world is polio free, we should keep all peoples of the world vaccinated so we don't lose ground in the eradication effort.

Second, until recently the U.S. (in accordance with World Health Organization recommendations) relied primarily on oral polio vaccine (OPV). This vaccine, containing live, weakened poliovirus, is highly effective, but it actually caused some cases of polio. So as of January 2000, OPV is no longer recommended except in limited situations. Instead, inactivated polio vaccine (IPV), the shot containing killed poliovirus, is recommended for the full series.

**Figure 10-1**
## GLOBAL DISTRIBUTION OF POLIO

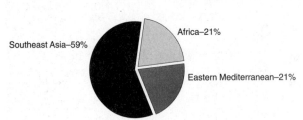

Southeast Asia–59%

Africa–21%

Eastern Mediterranean–21%

*Source:* Epidemiology and Prevention, *p. 102*

# THE POLIO DISEASE

## What is polio, and how is it spread?

Polio, also known as poliomyelitis, attacks cells in the spinal cord and brain stem. When nerves in these areas are destroyed, the muscles can no longer move; the person is paralyzed. The affected muscles shrink, or atrophy, and the limbs look shriveled (see Figure 10-2).

Although the virus most often attacks the nerves for arm or leg muscles, it can also affect other nerves, such as those for the diaphragm, the muscles used for breathing. Before the vaccine, entire wards were filled with polio patients who had to be kept alive by iron lung machines (see Figure 10-3).

The only way to catch the wild polio virus is from another person, but the virus is highly contagious. If one person in the household is infected, nearly all the nonimmunized children and adults in the family will also become infected. Poliovirus infection is most common in the summer in temperate climates.

Not everyone who is infected with poliovirus becomes paralyzed or dies. In fact, about 95 percent of all persons infected with polio have no symptoms. They are walking around among their healthy friends and family with no signs of the hidden danger. But their stools are passing poliovirus.

Fecal contamination can be found on many surfaces, especially in daycare centers. When a healthy person eats without having washed hands after changing diapers or when an infant or toddler explores her world tongue first, stool infected with poliovirus enters that person's mouth.

The viruses reproduce in the throat and intestines and then invade the lymph nodes and the bloodstream. Once in the bloodstream,

**Figure 10-2**
**POLIO**

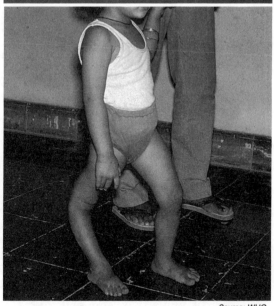

*Source: WHO*

· · · · · · · · · · · · · · · · · · · · · · · · · · · · · · · · · · · · · · · · · · · · · · · · · · · · · · · ·

**Figure 10-3**
**POLIO (the Drinker respirator ward, 1952)**

· · · · · · · · · · · · · · · · · · · · · · · · · · · · · · · · · · · · · · · · · · · · · · · · · · · · · · · ·

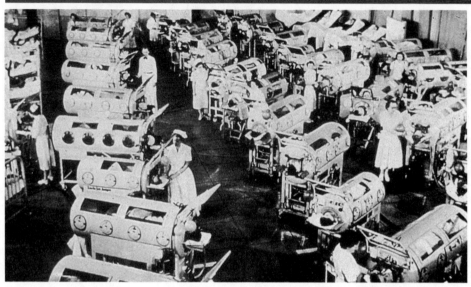

*Source: CDC*

they travel to the central nervous system where they destroy the brain stem and spinal nerves and cause symptoms such as weakness or increased or abnormal sensations. Before infected persons begin to show signs of nerve damage, though, they often have a minor, nonspecific illness that may include sore throat, fever, or nausea.

## IT HAPPENED TO DAVID

David Salamone contracted polio from the oral polio vaccine. John, David's father, says his son was perfectly healthy before receiving a second dose of live polio vaccine when David was 5 months old. Within hours of the vaccine his boy developed a fever, the next day a rash. Within weeks young David had lost the use of his body from the waist down.

"We cried for many nights," John recalls. The parents' grief turned to anger, and they began to ask, "Why did this have to happen?" Later tests revealed David had an undiagnosed immune deficiency, which made him especially vulnerable to the live vaccine.

David's condition has improved. Although his atrophied right leg remains in a brace, and the polio continues to affect his fine motor skills, he and his family feel lucky. Many victims of vaccine-associated paralytic polio don't fare as well.

John Salamone says he wishes government recommendations had changed to an all-IPV schedule a lot sooner: "It should have happened a decade or more ago."

## THE POLIO VACCINE

### What are the polio vaccines, and how effective are they?

In 1955, the first polio vaccine was licensed, after having been developed by Jonas Salk and his associates. It was called IPV, for inactivated polio vaccine, because it was comprised entirely of poliovirus that was killed, or inactivated by, formalin. In 1987, an improved version of IPV was licensed, and this is the version used today. But another form of the vaccine was to become the foundation of the effort to eradicate polio from the world.

**Inactivated Polio Vaccine (IPV).** After just two injections of IPV, 90 percent of people are immune to poliovirus and after three injections, 99 percent are immune. But IPV may not be effective for a lifetime. In France, which has relied primarily on IPV for years, adults receive boosters. One reason the U.S. is now willing to use IPV exclusively—aside from the risks associated with OPV—is that health officials are confident that we won't need to be immune in 10 years: the virus will have been eradicated by then.

**Oral Polio Vaccine (OPV).** Oral polio vaccine, or OPV, was developed by Dr. Albert Sabin and associates and licensed in 1961. The viruses in this vaccine are alive and rapidly reproduce in a person's intestines. This prompts the person's immune system to produce antibodies that protect from both the vaccine and the wild forms of the virus. After even one dose of OPV, 50 percent of persons are immune to polio, and after three doses, 95 percent are immune. Protection lasts for a lifetime after a full series of four doses.

OPV became the workhorse of the worldwide polio eradication program, almost entirely replacing IPV from the time it became available. Because it could be given without a needle or specially trained healthcare personnel, OPV has been used to painlessly vaccinate millions of children even in remote, impoverished areas of the globe.

Unfortunately, in rare instances OPV actually caused poliomyelitis in some of those persons who received it. For this reason, OPV is no longer recommended for routine use in the United States.

In the U. S., OPV is recommended now only in the following situations:

✣ When a child who is not immunized will be leaving the United States in less than four weeks for a place where polio is still active;

✣ When the parent of a child who already received two doses of IPV refuses further IPV injections for the child despite understanding the minimal risks; and

✣ As part of a mass immunization campaign to control an outbreak of wild polio.

A stockpile of OPV will be maintained in case of outbreaks, but the manufacturer no longer produces OPV for use in the U.S.

## Who should get polio vaccine and when?

The AAP and ACIP now recommend that only IPV be used for routine vaccination against polio in the U.S. From 1963 until 1996, OPV was used almost exclusively in the U.S. From 1996 through 1999, children usually received two doses of IPV and then two of OPV. But beginning in January 2000, children were recommended to receive all four doses of polio vaccine in IPV form. The recommended age for the four doses are 2 months, 4 months, between 6 and 18 months, and before beginning school.

Under normal circumstances, persons aged 18 and older don't need polio vaccine in the U.S. because they are probably already immune and have little chance of coming in contact with poliovirus. However, adults, including pregnant women, do need polio vaccine if they

✣ Plan to travel to a polio-infected area,

✣ Handle lab specimens that may contain poliovirus,

✣ Are in close contact with patients who may be shedding poliovirus in their stool, or

✛ Live in a community where there is a polio outbreak.

If you need polio vaccine, talk to your healthcare provider about which form of vaccine is right for you. (See Table 10-1.)

## Who should *not* get the vaccine?

IPV should not be used if the child or adult has the following conditions:

✛ Serious allergy such as hives or difficulty breathing after a previous vaccine dose or vaccine component. IPV contains minute amounts of antibiotics (such as streptomycin, neomycin, and polymyxin B).

✛ A moderate or severe illness that your healthcare provider believes will be more complicated to manage if the vaccine is used. In this case wait until the illness has ended.

**Table 10-1**

**RECOMMENDATIONS FOR ADULTS AT INCREASED RISK OF EXPOSURE TO POLIOVIRUS**

| Polio vaccine received in the past | Vaccine recommended now |
| --- | --- |
| ✛ Full series of OPV or IPV | One more dose of OPV or IPV |
| ✛ Incomplete series of OPV or IPV | As many doses as needed to complete the series |
| ✛ None | Three doses of IPV Doses #1 and #2 separated by 4 to 8 weeks Doses #2 and #3 separated by 6 to 12 months (If protection will be needed in less than a month, use one dose of OPV or IPV.) |

*Source: MMWR 46: RR-3 (1997)*

## What are the vaccine risks and side effects?

Allergic reactions can occur after any vaccine. Among people receiving IPV, minor pain or redness at the injection site is reported in 13 percent and fever of 102 degrees Fahrenheit or higher in 38 percent of the cases.

OPV in rare cases can cause paralysis. This happens when reproduction of the live virus contained in OPV goes awry. Instead of being an exact copy of its parent virus, the offspring virus is like the wild poliovirus and can cause paralytic disease that is every bit as bad as paralytic polio from the wild virus. From 1980 to 1994, 125 people in the U.S.—roughly 1 case for every 2.4 million doses of OPV—developed vaccine-associated paralytic polio, or VAPP. About a third of these victims were previously healthy children who received OPV; about a third were previously healthy but not immunized family members and friends of children who received OPV; and the remaining third were people who were immuno-compromised.

## What are additional historical controversies?

**SV40.** Simian virus (or SV) 40 is a virus found in the kidney cells of monkeys. Vaccine manufacturing methods did not include a test for SV40 until 1961, so some experimental OPV and fully licensed IPV received by as many as 30 million Americans between 1954 and 1962 may have contained SV40. SV40 can cause cancer in lab animals, and some of its DNA sequences have been found in rare human tumors (although some researchers dispute this). Studies in the U.S. and Sweden, however, have shown that cancer rates did not increase among people who could have been exposed to SV40. Since 1961, manufacturers have been required to test for SV40 and destroy contaminated vaccine lots. Also, the source of monkey cells was changed to a species that does not harbor SV40.

**The Cutter Incident.** In April 1955, just months after 400,000 children, mostly first and second graders, were given the IPV made by Cutter Laboratories, 360 of them became paralyzed. The poliovirus had not been fully killed before the children were given the immunization. The disaster led to more stringent guidelines for the manufacturing and testing of polio vaccine. Since then, not a single case has been reported of a child contracting polio after receiving IPV.

## WHAT OTHER QUESTIONS DO PARENTS ASK?

*Q: My child already received one OPV dose. Should we switch to IPV for the rest of the series?*

Yes. Current recommendations call for an all-IPV schedule, and there is no harm in switching from OPV to IPV.

*Q: Why should my child get the polio shot if there isn't any polio in the Western Hemisphere?*

There are three reasons for your child to receive polio vaccine. First, the vaccine prevents polio disease. Although no wild polio disease has originated in the U.S. since 1979 or in the Western Hemisphere since 1991, until the disease is eradicated in the rest of the world it remains just a plane ride away.

Second, giving your child IPV protects against any effect from poliovirus shed in the stool of children who may have received live oral polio vaccine.

Third, continued use of this vaccine will prevent spread of the disease and help the efforts to eradicate the disease. After the world has been certified to be polio free, no one will need polio vaccine anymore, just as we no longer need smallpox vaccine.

*Q: Why did the U.S. government take so long to change the recommendations when they knew OPV could cause paralytic polio?*

There was a great debate over moving away from primary reliance on OPV. OPV gave children immediate, long-term, painless, and inexpensive protection from polio. The key was that OPV produced antibodies in the intestines, so if someone swallowed wild poliovirus, it could not set up residence in the child's system. Public health experts feared that people vaccinated with IPV could carry wild polio in their gut and spread it to unvaccinated people. There was also concern that other countries would follow the U.S. and move away from OPV, jeopardizing the eradication effort.

*Q: Can my child infect others with polio after he receives the inactivated form of the vaccine?*

No. IPV does not contain any living material, so it cannot cause infection in the people who receive it or the people in close contact with them.

*Q: What is post-polio syndrome?*

Thirty to 40 years after having paralytic polio, some people may develop post-polio syndrome. It is believed to occur because of the gradual reduction of nervous system cells during aging, which unmasks nerve damage from the original polio infection years before. The signs and symptoms include new muscle pain, and new or worsened muscle weakness. Women are more likely than men to get post-polio syndrome, and people with permanent residual weakness are more likely to get it than those who had completely recovered. The risk of post-polio syndrome also increases as more time elapses after the original infection. It is not a flare-up of the polio infection, and there is no danger to household members that polio will be spread.

Support groups have formed to help people with post-polio syndrome and their families. These include the following:

⊹ International Polio Network (314-534-0475)

⊹ March of Dimes Birth Defects Foundation National Headquarters, Program Services (914-428-7100)

⊹ Roosevelt Warm Springs Institute (706-655-5000)

*Q: How do we know that there is no wild polio in the U.S.?*

The National Immunization Program of the CDC, in conjunction with state and local health authorities, monitors the U.S. for cases of paralysis that might be poliomyelitis. Cases should be reported to state and local health authorities and to the CDC (404-639-8255).

*Q: Did the polio vaccine cause the AIDS epidemic?*

In his book *The River: A Journey to the Source of HIV and AIDS,* British journalist Edward Hooper hypothesizes that the virus that causes AIDS originally passed from chimpanzees to humans during the testing of OPV. He argues that the experimental vaccine was produced with chimpanzee tissues infected with an HIV-related monkey virus, though scientists were unaware of the contamination. The contaminated vaccine was given to children in an area of Africa that was then the Belgian Congo (now Burundi, the Congo, and Rwanda) and today is considered the center of the AIDS epidemic.

In a December 7, 1999, letter to the *New York Times,* Drs. Stanley Plotkin and Hilary Koprowski, the physicians who conducted the implicated trials, state "No chimpanzee tissues were used by us for polio vaccine production." They point out that "Two independent analyses of the probable timing of the crossover of HIV from chimpanzees into humans give dates far earlier than 1957–1959, the years in which our polio vaccine was used in the Congo."

Scientists at the CDC also point out that it is unlikely such a contaminant virus could survive freezing and thawing cycles used in OPV preparation, or the enzymes and acids in the human mouth and stomach. Previous testing of one of the original experimental OPV lots showed no sign of an HIV-related virus, but in November 1999, the Wistar Institute, which developed the vaccine, announced that it would allow two independent laboratories to test both original lots to reach a definitive conclusion.

## WHAT DOES THE FUTURE HOLD?

**The eradication of polio.** When polio vaccine became available, parents clamored to get it for their children. Since 1985, the nations of North and South America have worked together to eliminate polio, so that by 1991 the Western Hemisphere saw its last case of wild polio. In 2000, the World Health Assembly resolved to eradicate polio by 2005. Great progress is being made. In 1999, fifty countries were infected by polio; by early 2000 the number of infected countries had dropped to thirty. In 2000, China became certified as polio free.

In spite of conflict within and among nations, there has been tremendous cooperation in the work of eliminating polio. In Central America, cease-fires have even been arranged during wars to ensure full vaccination of children. Similar efforts have been made in Afghanistan and parts of Africa. With the help of Rotary International, global eradication of poliovirus is expected early in the twenty-first century.

**Combination vaccines with polio.** Canada and Mexico already have licensed combination vaccines that include IPV and four other vaccines. These combination vaccines decrease the number of injections needed. Not too far in the future, the FDA may license such a product for use in the U.S.

*Medicine, the only profession that labors incessantly to destroy the reason for its own existence.*

—Lord Bryce

# Chapter 11

# Hib Vaccine

The CDC estimates that before the Hib (*Haemophilus influenzae* type b) vaccine was licensed in 1985, each year about 20,000 children in the U.S. developed Hib disease, and about 500 children died of it. Nearly all of these patients were younger than 5 years old. Many of those who survived were left blind, deaf, learning disabled, or permanently brain damaged. In fact, before the vaccine, this disease caused the most common form of mental retardation acquired after birth.

Hib vaccine began to be used in the late 1980s. By 1998, only 228 children caught Hib disease, a decline of almost 99 percent. (See Figure 11-1.)

Despite its name, *Haemophilus influenzae* type b is not related to influenza. The doctor who named the disease in the late 1800s confused it with the influenza that his patient also had. The real nature of Hib was not clarified until the 1930s.

Because Hib often causes a form of meningitis, its vaccine has been called "the meningitis vaccine." But meningitis has many different causes and forms, which we discuss here and in Chapter 15, Pneumococcus, and in Chapter 17, Meningococcus.

## THE HIB DISEASE

### What is Hib, and how is it spread?

The Hib bacteria travel through the bloodstream and settle in parts of the body. Most often they settle in the brain, causing bacterial meningitis. Meningitis and other infections caused by Hib are addressed below (see also Figure 11-2):

✚ **Meningitis** is an infection of the outer lining of the brain. Signs of bacterial meningitis initially are a high fever, irritability, and decreased appetite, and later, decreased mental alertness and a stiff neck. About 50 to 65 percent of Hib cases are in the form of meningitis. Of those children who get Hib meningitis, 2 to 5 percent will die of it, even if they are treated quickly. Of those who live, 15 to 30 percent will develop seizures, deafness, or mental retardation.

✚ **Epiglottitis** is an infection of the tissue flap at the base of the throat where the windpipe (trachea) meets the food pipe (esophagus). Swelling could lead to blockage of the airway, which can be fatal if not treated immediately. Children with epiglottitis make a gasping sound with each attempt to inhale. They are anxious looking and they instinctively tend to lean forward to get in the best position to keep from closing off their airway.

✚ **Pneumonia** is an infection of the lungs. Hib pneumonia can be very severe. Signs and symptoms include fever, cough, and, if untreated, difficulty getting enough oxygen into the lungs.

✚ **Osteomyelitis** is an infection of the bone, which can destroy the bone. If the infection gets to the growth

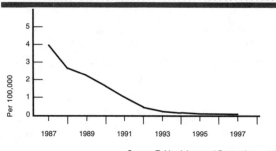

**Figure 11-1**

**CASES OF INVASIVE HIB DISEASE AMONG CHILDREN UNDER 5 YEARS OLD, 1987–1997**

*Source: Epidemiology and Prevention, p. 123*

plate, the bone stops growing, and the limb becomes
deformed. Signs and symp-
toms are fever, redness,
swelling, and pain in the
limb.

✛ **Septic arthritis** is an infection of a joint, which can
destroy the joint. Signs and
symptoms are fever, redness,
swelling, and pain in the
joint.

**Figure 11-2**
## MANIFESTATIONS OF HIB

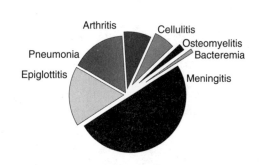

Source: Epidemiology and Prevention, p. 121

✛ **Cellulitis** is an infection of the skin, often of the head, face, or
neck. This is not life- or limb-threatening in itself, but Hib in the
bloodstream can spread to other sites, including the meninges
surrounding the brain. Signs and symptoms include fever, redness, swelling, and pain at the site of infection.

✛ **Bacteremia** is an infection in the bloodstream. The primary
symptom is fever. Like cellulitis, bacteremia's danger is that Hib
in the bloodstream can spread to other sites, including the
meninges of the brain.

Hib germs spread from person to person, probably by small respiratory
droplets. They set up residence in a person's nose and/or throat and may
stay there briefly or for months. Some children may carry the germ around
for months without getting sick, while other children might get sick immediately as the bacteria invade the bloodstream and cause devastating effects.
Most of the persons who contract Hib disease are infants, usually around 6
to 7 months of age.

Few children catch Hib disease beyond 5 years of age. Invasive Hib is
not very contagious. Only 3 out of 1,000 people in close contact with a
child who has invasive Hib will develop the disease. Certain conditions put
a person at higher risk for getting Hib disease, such as the following:

✛ Close contact with other children. More children get Hib disease if they have school-aged siblings or attend daycare. Once one member of a household contracts Hib, the risk of others in the household catching it is about 600 times higher than it is in the general population.

✛ Race or ethnicity. More Blacks, Hispanics, and Native Americans than Caucasians get Hib disease.

✛ Some chronic diseases. Sickle-cell anemia, cancer, and antibody deficiency conditions lead to an increased risk.

✛ Sex. More males than females get Hib disease.

## Is Hib still a threat?

The vaccine reduces the proportion of children who carry Hib bacteria in their nose and throats, so the more children who are vaccinated, the fewer children who can spread the germ. In 1998, 93 percent of children received three doses of Hib vaccine by 2 years of age, making the U.S. a little safer for other children. However, even though the vaccine provides personal protection from invasive Hib disease, some vaccinated children still carry and spread Hib bacteria, so it remains a threat.

### It Happened to Sarah

Peggy Archer, mother of three and a nurse from Michigan, will always regret not giving her young daughter the Hib vaccine on schedule. And still she acknowledges that Sarah "probably would not have survived had I not used my nursing instinct."

The terrible ordeal began not long after Peggy noticed 2-year-old Sarah wasn't feeling well. Peggy thought it was "your basic childhood fever and upper respiratory illness." But it didn't go away. Within days, Sarah's breathing became "labored, she started to drool, and I knew we were in trouble." By the time they got to the hospital, Sarah's airway was so swollen that doctors had a difficult time intubating her. She couldn't swallow. She couldn't breathe.

Peggy describes those moments as being filled with "terror, absolute terror. The scariest couple of hours I've ever had in my life." She says that when they took her daughter in, "I knew we had waited too long, and they might not be able to save her. That was the worst, not knowing if I would ever get her back."

The doctor confirmed that Sarah had been infected with the Hib bacteria. One doctor even chided Peggy saying, "Well, this wouldn't have happened if you had gotten the Hib vaccine."

Peggy responds, "I was just devastated. I consider myself a good mom."

Sarah recovered. Today she is a healthy 13 year old with no memory of her brush with death. Still, when Peggy describes what happened years ago, she is filled with emotion. "The vaccine was new. I knew she needed it. It was on my list of things to do. It just didn't get done in time."

"I would never want another parent to experience what I experienced," Peggy concludes. "I remember thinking, 'Gee, if I had just gotten her the shot, she wouldn't have gone through all this.' I could have prevented this torture."

Peggy's two younger children received all their vaccines, including Hib, right on schedule.

---

## THE Hib VACCINE

### What is the Hib vaccine, and how effective is it?

The first Hib vaccine was licensed in 1985, but it did not protect children younger than 18 months old, who are most vulnerable to the disease. An improved version of the vaccine was licensed in 1987, but that still was not very effective for infants. Since 1990, the FDA has licensed four manufacturers to produce Hib vaccines that are effective in children as young as 6 weeks old. The Hib vaccines are effective in 95 percent or more of the children who receive the full series.

## Who should get Hib vaccine and when?

**Young children.** Hib vaccine is recommended for most children who have not yet reached their fifth birthday. Most brands of Hib vaccine are given as injections at 2, 4, 6, and 12 to 15 months of age. If the Hib vaccine made by Merck is used for all doses, only three doses are necessary, and these should be given at 2, 4, and 12 to 15 months of age. It's fine if different brands are given for different doses, but if this is done, then four shots are needed to complete the series.

**Other children and adults.** Most people who are more than 5 years old do not need Hib vaccine unless they have sickle-cell anemia, problems with their spleen, or a weakened immune system.

## Who should *not* get the vaccine?

Hib vaccine should not be given to your child if he or she

✛ Is less than 6 weeks old or has already passed the fifth birthday,

✛ Had a serious allergic reaction to a prior dose of Hib vaccine, or

✛ Has a moderate to severe illness. If this is the case, the vaccine should be given without fail when the child is feeling better.

## What are the vaccine risks and side effects?

The Hib vaccine has a good safety record. But allergic reactions can occur after any vaccine. These are the other risks and side effects that have been known to occur after Hib vaccines.

✛ Minor pain, swelling, or redness at the injection site may begin soon after the shot and usually resolves within a day. Anywhere between 10 and 15 percent of children will experience these symptoms.

✛ Fever or irritability may begin within a few hours of vaccination and usually resolves within a day or two. About 2 percent of children will experience this.

## WHAT OTHER QUESTIONS DO PARENTS ASK?

*Q: Does Hib vaccine cause diabetes?*

No. The National Institutes of Allergy and Infectious Diseases, a U.S. federal agency, held a meeting of experts in May 1998 to debate the diabetes issue. They concluded that existing studies in humans do not indicate an increase in diabetes due to vaccines or the timing of vaccination.

*Q: Are those vaccinated more susceptible to Hib meningitis in the first week following vaccination?*

No. The risk of Hib disease is not increased in the weeks following vaccination with a modern Hib vaccine. The vaccine should not be expected to work immediately, however.

*Q: Is it safe for parents not to have their child vaccinated if they stay home with the child during the first 12 to 18 months when the disease most often occurs?*

No statistic is available on the risk of Hib disease in a child who is otherwise healthy, has no siblings, and is not in close or prolonged contact with other children. Such a child would have a lower risk than those with siblings or playmates, but safety cannot be guaranteed, of course.

*Q: A child in my son's daycare developed Hib disease. My child has definitely received all his vaccines. Should he also take antibiotics?*

No. Children who are fully vaccinated do not need antibiotics in such cases. But do make sure someone has reported this case to the local or state health department.

## WHAT DOES THE FUTURE HOLD?

Hib vaccine will probably be added to an increasingly large number of combination vaccines (such as DTaP plus Hib plus IPV), but is is impossible to predict when these combination vaccines will be licensed for use in the United States. These combinations will make it possible for children to receive fewer injections and yet get the same powerful protection.

*Love iz like the meazles; we kant have it bad but onst, and the later in life we have it the tuffer it goes with us.*

—Josh Billings [Henry Wheeler Shaw]

# Chapter 12

# MMR Vaccine:
## Measles, Mumps, and Rubella

We have entered a remarkable era in the history of measles. New evidence suggests that this highly contagious disease, once considered more dreaded than smallpox, no longer circulates in the United States. Small numbers of cases are imported from economically advantaged nations (such as Germany and Japan), as well as such countries as China, Cyprus, Croatia, and Zimbabwe, but disease has reached a record low. This public health success has occurred because vaccination with one dose of measles vaccine is at a record high and most U.S. students live in states that require them to receive a second dose.

Even with this success, MMR, the vaccine that offers protection against measles, mumps, and rubella, is controversial. Much of this controversy centers on the suggestion that MMR is associated with a modern American epidemic: autism (see page 36). Parents, frightened by the allegations, are questioning the value of the measles vaccine at the same time that public health officials have begun to develop plans for the global elimination of measles, rubella, and one of the few known causes of autism, congenital rubella.

## MEASLES

Through the mid-1960s, virtually everyone got measles. It was an expected life event, as chickenpox was until recently. Before a measles vaccine was licensed in 1963, each year in the United States as many as 4 million people got sick from the disease and 1,000 people died. More than 50 percent of the population caught the measles by age 6, and more than 90 percent by age 15. After measles vaccine was licensed in 1963, the number of measles cases in the U.S. dropped by 90 percent in five years. By 1998, because of the widespread use of MMR vaccine, a record low of 100 measles cases and no deaths were reported.

Measles is no longer circulating in the United States, but it is rampant in other parts of the world today. According to Dr. Walter Orenstein, Director of the National Immunization Program of the CDC, measles "could return at any time should immunization levels drop." In the not-so-distant past (1989–91) when immunization levels were low, a measles outbreak in the U.S. resulted in 53,632 cases and 123 deaths. Ninety percent of those who died had never received the measles vaccine. (See Figure 12-1.)

### What is measles, and how is it spread?

Measles is a virus that causes fever that lasts for a couple days, followed by a cough, runny nose, and pink eye. A rash starts on the face and upper neck, spreads down the back and trunk, then extends to the arms and hands, as well as the legs and feet (Figure 12-2). After about five days, the rash fades in the same order it appeared.

Measles itself is unpleasant, but the complications are dangerous. Six to 8 percent of people who contract measles will then get pneumonia, ear infection, or diarrhea. One out of 1,000 will develop inflammation of the brain, and 2 out of 1,000 will die. (See Figures 12-3 A & B.)

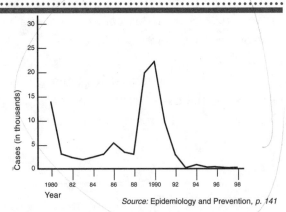

**Figure 12-1**
**MEASLES IN THE UNITED STATES, 1980–1998**

Cases (in thousands)

Year

*Source:* Epidemiology and Prevention, p. 141

In countries where malnutrition and vitamin A deficiency are prevalent, measles has been known to kill as many as one out of four people. It is the leading cause of blindness among African children.

If a pregnant woman catches measles, her fetus is at risk of prematurity, low birth weight, and even death. Birth defects have been reported, but it is unclear if measles was the direct cause.

Measles can be spread from four days before to four days after the rash. The measles virus resides in the mucus in the nose and throat of infected people. When they sneeze or cough, droplets spray into the air. The droplets of infected mucus can land in other persons' noses or throats when they inhale, mouth a toy, or put their fingers in their mouth or nose after handling an infected surface. The virus remains active and contagious on infected surfaces for two hours.

**Figure 12-2**
## MEASLES (DAY 4)

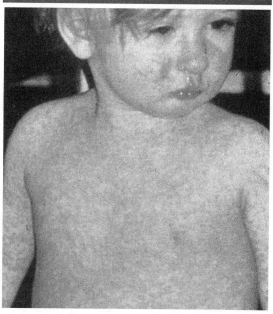

*Source: CDC*

**Figure 12-3A**
## MEASLES COMPLICATIONS

| CONDITION | PERCENT REPORTED |
| --- | --- |
| Any complication* | 29 |
| Diarrhea | 8 |
| Otitis media | 7 |
| Pneumonia | 6 |
| Encephalitis | 0.1 |
| Death | 0.2 |
| Hospitalization | 18 |

*Includes hospitalization; data from 1985 to 1992

*Source:* Epidemiology and Prevention, *p. 137*

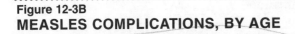

**Figure 12-3B**
## MEASLES COMPLICATIONS, BY AGE

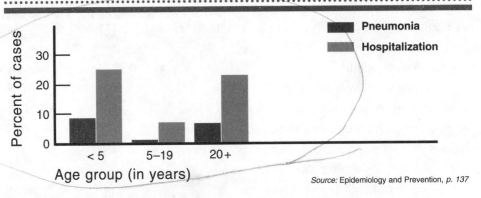

*Source:* Epidemiology and Prevention, *p. 137*

Although the virus is no longer constantly circulating in the U.S., outbreaks due to importation continue to occur. In August 1999, a minister traveling abroad brought measles home to the United States, ultimately infecting at least 13 people. The ordeal began when the 36-year-old minister from Bedford County, Virginia, flew to Rome, then on to Bahrain, Muscat, Nairobi, and Abu Dhabi. After returning home, he spoke at several church services before developing fever, a sore throat, and a cough. Soon all three of his unvaccinated children, ages 2 to 8, became ill with the measles. Five church members contracted the measles, too. One of them, a 30-year-old woman, was hospitalized and there transmitted the virus to two healthcare workers. A 13-month-old boy infected at church transmitted the virus to his 36-year-old uncle. The uncle gave the virus to an 18 month old and to his brother. In all, 13 people ended up sick because they were unprotected and exposed to the measles virus that had been brought in from another country. Most cases of measles in the U.S. now result from international travel or because of spreading from imported cases.

People of any age, sex, race, or ethnicity can catch measles. If one person has it, then 90 percent of their susceptible close contacts will get it, too.

## IT HAPPENED TO AARON

Becki Chottiner of Livonia, Michigan, is angry with parents who don't immunize their children. She believes one such parent is to blame for a measles outbreak that left her sick and nearly took her son's life.

In May 1998, just a month before her 11-month-old son Aaron was due for his <u>MMR vaccine</u>, he came home from daycare with red, watery eyes, a cough, and mild fever. Soon he developed a rash behind his ears. A young doctor unfamiliar with measles diagnosed Aaron as having "a nonspecific viral illness." Despite a rash and double ear infection, the doctor said Aaron would be fine. But he was not.

Becki said lesions inside his mouth made it difficult for Aaron to eat or sleep. By that time the rash covered his entire body. For a second time she and her son were told to sit in a crowded waiting room. After being tested for measles, reassured, and sent home yet again, Aaron began coughing up his food and vomiting everything he drank. While waiting for tests to confirm measles, Becki too began to feel achy and feverish. Finally an epidemiologist from the Michigan Department of Community Health drove to her house and conducted tests confirming that she, like her son, had measles. Becki suspects the single dose of MMR she received as a child had not adequately protected her—which is why children today are given a second dose.

Becki recovered, but young Aaron continued to spike a high fever and cough up food. "We will never forget how sick he was, just lying on the floor because he couldn't do anything else," she recalls. Finally a chest X ray revealed pneumonia in his right lung. Once hospitalized, Becki says, he had two operations, but part of his lung collapsed. That's when, Becki says, "it hit me how serious it was. There was actually the chance we could lose him over something as stupid as the measles."

While Aaron now has long been free of measles, other respiratory ailments continue to plague him. To protect him, the entire family gets flu shots every year. They continue to watch Aaron each day. "He's started to grow again," Becki adds. "He seems to be doing better, but we'll have to see." Becki has cut her work schedule to part time to care for him, since his colds often lead to complications, as Aaron has "chronic recurrent pneumonia."

Becki is relieved her son is alive. But she is also angry. She is not mad about the $20,000 in hospital bills. She doesn't blame the doctors for not knowing her son had measles, but she does blame some anonymous caregiver whose apparent decision not to vaccinate threatened her family.

"One person who wasn't immunized made several babies sick with the disease, and three of them were hospitalized." Becki continues, "We have an obligation to consider not only our own children, but all the children they come into contact with. We do have to consider the good of the community."

## MUMPS

Until the late 1960s, mumps was not as common as measles, but was still a well-known disease. In 1964, three years before the first mumps vaccine was licensed, an estimated 212,000 people in the U.S. got the disease. By 1998, thanks to the vaccine, only 606 cases were reported.

### What is mumps, and how is it spread?

The mumps virus is spread the same way as measles, by particles of mucus in the air or on surfaces, but mumps is not as contagious as measles. Mumps is most common in children 5 to 19 years old.

**Figure 12-4**
**MUMPS**

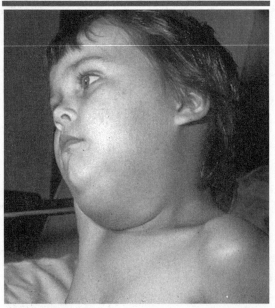

Source: CDC

Mumps often causes saliva glands to swell for a week to ten days (Figure 12-4). Before the swelling begins, the infected person may have muscle aches, low-grade fever, decreased appetite, headache, and a general feeling of malaise. Twenty percent of people who are infected with the mumps virus don't even know it, and another 40 to 50 percent have a mild illness that no one suspects is mumps.

Like measles, the complications are the worst part. The chief complications of mumps are inflammation of the central nervous system (meningitis occurs in up to 15 percent of patients with mumps, but usually resolves without permanent deficits); inflammation of the testicles (in 20 to 50 percent of males who get mumps any time after puberty) or ovaries (in 5 percent of females who get mumps after puberty); deafness, usually on one side; and, in rare occasions, death.

More than 600 cases of mumps were reported in the U.S. in 1998. Although mumps has decreased by 99.7 percent since the mid-1960s, it's not history yet.

## RUBELLA (GERMAN MEASLES)

Rubella, often known as German measles, was once as common as childhood itself. In the 1964–65 outbreak of rubella, 12.5 million Americans contracted the disease. Rubella is a fairly minor disease, but it can be devastating or fatal to a developing fetus. Unfortunately, many of the patients were pregnant women, so about 11,000 fetuses died from spontaneous and therapeutic abortions, and 20,000 infants were born with permanent disabilities such as deafness, blindness, or mental retardation. By 1998, thanks to vaccinations, only 364 cases of rubella and 7 cases of fetal damage from rubella were reported. All cases of rubella fetal damage occurred in children of women born outside the U.S. in countries that don't routinely use rubella vaccine.

**Figure 12-5**
**RUBELLA (adolescent)**

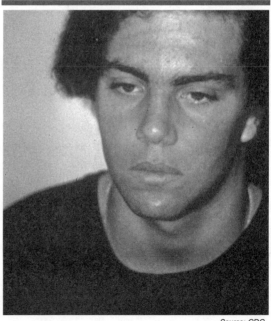

Source: CDC

### What is rubella, and how is it spread?

Rubella is a virus that spreads the same way as measles, but rubella is not as contagious as measles. People who are infected by rubella, whether or not they have symptoms, spread the virus.

Rubella often has no symptoms. When signs and symptoms do appear, young children will usually first have a rash; older children and adults may develop an illness like a common cold plus swollen glands in the head and neck, then the rash (Figure 12-5).

A few complications of this disease are a bit more worrisome. Adults (up to 70 percent of women) often have joint pain and swelling that may last up to a month. Brain inflammation occurs in 1 out of 5,000 infected people, more often in women. Bleeding within the digestive system, the brain, or the kidneys occurs in 1 out of 3,000 infected people, more often among children. Fortunately, most patients recover from such bleeding disorders in a matter of days to months.

The most dreaded complication occurs in fetuses of pregnant women who become infected with rubella early in the pregnancy. An infant with congenital rubella syndrome (CRS) may develop deafness, cataracts, a wide range of heart defects, and/or mental retardation, as well as bone, liver, and spleen abnormalities. As the child grows, problems may become apparent such as learning disabilities, diabetes, or a degenerative brain disease that leads to death. Preventing the devastation caused by congenital rubella syndrome is at the heart of the rubella vaccination program.

Before the vaccine, the highest proportion of people who contracted rubella were children. In recent years, as the number of persons infected has plummeted, the distribution has shifted dramatically. In 1997, more than 75 percent of the 161 persons who caught rubella in the U.S. were 20 to 39 years old. Most of them were born in countries where rubella vaccine is not used routinely (even Mexico did not use rubella vaccine until 1998). Rubella remains a threat because it is easily imported to the U.S.

## THE MMR VACCINE

### What is the MMR vaccine, and how effective is it?

Two kinds of measles vaccines were first licensed in 1963. In 1967, the "killed" vaccine was found to be ineffective and was removed from the market. (Note: If you were vaccinated only once between 1963 and 1967 and you don't know which vaccine you received, talk to your healthcare provider about getting MMR.) The live vaccine, the other original vaccine, has been improved several times over the years. The strain of vaccine virus in use now was licensed in 1968.

Similarly, a mumps vaccine was developed in 1948, but it produced only short-term immunity so it was withdrawn from the market in the mid-1970s. The vaccine currently in use was licensed in 1967. Three rubella vaccines were licensed in 1969, but the one in use today in the United States was licensed in 1979.

Measles, mumps, and rubella vaccines were first licensed as a combination in 1971. The MMR used today in the U.S. contains the safest and most effective of each of the vaccines.

## Who should get MMR vaccine and when?

**Children.** Children should be given one dose of MMR on or after the first birthday. The second dose is recommended before the start of kindergarten. About 95 percent of the children who receive one dose of MMR at 12 months of age become immune, and after two doses about 99.7 percent of children become immune. Two doses are also recommended for children and adolescents who were not vaccinated as infants.

**Adults.** Adults born after 1956 should receive at least one dose of MMR unless they are immune to measles, mumps, and rubella. Adults at increased risk (such as persons traveling abroad, attending college, or working at a healthcare facility) should have received two doses of MMR, including the doses received as children.

Also, if a woman who was born before 1957 could become pregnant, she should be sure that she is immune to rubella. That can be done with a blood test or a dose of rubella vaccine (preferably given as MMR). She also should make sure not to become pregnant for three months after receiving the rubella vaccination.

## Who should *not* get the vaccine?

MMR should *not* be given to anyone who has the following conditions:

✛ A serious allergic reaction to a prior dose of MMR or to a prior exposure to its contents (such as gelatin, neomycin).

✛ A weakened immune system. People with HIV infection who don't have symptoms of AIDS may receive MMR. (MMR may be given to children with an immuno-deficient household member.)

✛ Pregnancy (but MMR may be given to children with a pregnant household member).

✛ A moderate to severe illness. If this is the case, the vaccine should be given without fail when the child is feeling better.

✛ Recent intake of a blood product that contains antibodies (such as immune globulin).

✛ Low platelet count. People who have had low platelet counts should talk to their healthcare provider about whether to get MMR or not. A decision needs to be made about whether the risk of the vaccine is greater or less than the risk of the diseases.

### What are the vaccine risks and side effects?

Allergic reactions could occur after any vaccine. These are the other risks and side effects that have been known to occur after MMR vaccine. Reactions more commonly appear after the first than after the second dose of vaccine.

✛ Fever or irritability may begin 7 to 12 days after vaccination; these symptoms usually resolve within a day or two. About 5 percent of susceptible children will develop a fever of 103 degrees or higher after the first dose.

✛ Rash is most likely to begin 7 to 10 days after vaccination and usually resolves within a few days. About 5 percent of susceptible people will experience this.

✛ Joint pain develops in about 25 percent of susceptible women after rubella vaccines, including MMR.

✛ Joint inflammation (redness, swelling, warmth, and pain) develops in about 10 percent of this group. Joint symptoms, which are usually mild, start 1 to 3 weeks after vaccination and last 1 to 21 days. Although some persons have questioned whether rubella vaccines caused long-term or recurring joint problems, recent data on the use of the currently licensed U.S. vaccine refutes this.

✛ Low platelet count may develop within two months of vaccination in about 1 out of 30,000 to 40,000 children. Because platelets help in blood clotting, physicians worry that this side effect will lead to bleeding, but it rarely does. (If you catch rubella or measles themselves, you are more likely to have bleeding than you would be after the vaccine, but even developing a bleeding disorder after the disease is rare.) This side effect seems to occur more frequently in persons who have had low platelet count in the past, whether from the first dose of MMR or from another disorder (such as ITP).

✛ Seizure occurs after 1 out of 3,000 doses of MMR. Some children have a seizure when they develop a fever. If a child, any siblings, or a parent has a history of seizures from a fever, then discuss preventing the fever with the child's healthcare provider.

✛ Brain inflammation, deafness, and testicular inflammation have been associated with mumps vaccines used in other countries. In 1993, a group of independent scientists at the Institute of Medicine (IOM) concluded that they did not have enough information to decide if the mumps vaccine licensed in the U.S. ever caused these side effects. If it did, the occurrences were very rare. Similarly, IOM did not have sufficient evidence to accept or reject a causal relation between MMR and Guillain-Barré syndrome, a paralyzing condition of nerves.

---

### IT HAPPENED TO ANNA

Fifteen-month-old Anna Coqliandro of Chesapeake, Virginia, had a rare, adverse reaction to MMR, according to her mother, Colette. Colette says she took the child in for a well-baby checkup and vaccines. The doctor gave Anna MMR in her thigh. Several days later, Colette noticed that Anna had a hard time with her fine motor skills. Also, Colette explains, Anna's "personality changed. She wanted me to hold her all the time. There was a hard knot at the injection site. She was fretful. Then she began falling."

The damage was slow and progressive. Six weeks after the vaccine, Anna stopped walking. Tests conducted by a neurologist showed swelling and lesions on Anna's brain. Anna had encephalitis. Colette thought she was "in the middle of a nightmare" when the doctor said, "your daughter has permanent brain damage." After additional tests, the neurologist concluded that Anna's encephalopathy was due to MMR.

At age 2, Anna could no longer speak or sit up. Doctors at Duke University Medical School conducted still more tests to rule out other causes. Colette says doctors there told her that Anna might die.

She watched her child receive MRI after MRI. She listened to her once-smiling, healthy daughter scream under the mammoth medical equipment. Colette stared out the hospital window. "For brief moments I thought about jumping out. I had thoughts of suicide." But "a little voice inside me said it's going to be okay. She [Anna] is going to need me." Later doctors told Colette, "Don't rule out a miracle, but Anna will never walk again."

Today, at age 11 as of this writing, Anna still cannot walk on her own. She has difficulty speaking and using her hands. While the brain damage affected her physical abilities, her intellect remains intact. Anna goes to school with other children her age. An A student, she is active in drama and was on the Internet when I asked to speak with her.

Anna says, "When I was really little, like 15 months old, I got a shot. My mom thought it would be good for me. I had a reaction and got brain damage. It wasn't my mother's fault."

Colette, who cherishes her daughter, feels blessed. "I don't take anything for granted." She urges other parents to "follow their gut feelings." With regard to vaccines, she says, "All parents have to make their own decisions."

Anna's family received damages from the National Injury Compensation Program. Serious reactions to MMR rarely occur.

## WHAT OTHER QUESTIONS DO PARENTS ASK?

Q: *Does MMR cause autism?*

No one knows for certain what causes autism, and research on autism is difficult since no one thoroughly understands what it is. Evidence suggests that what we now refer to as autism may be several different conditions. Autism does have different manifestations. For example, some autistic children developed normally at first and then had notable regression, while others had unusual behaviors even during infancy.

Recently, the National Institutes of Health have begun funding research on autism. Preliminary work from these and other studies suggest that MMR does not cause autism. For example, studies have shown that autism is about four times more common among boys than girls, but vaccination rates of MMR do not differ between boys and girls. A genetic cause has also been implicated by studies showing that if one identical twin is autistic, the other twin is at greatly increased risk for autism. Further, some studies have shown differences in brain structures of autistic children that develop in the first few weeks of fetal development.

One large study showed that unvaccinated children were as likely as vaccinated children to develop autism. Additional studies are further evaluating the relationship between autism and vaccination. (An excellent summary of the research to date can be found at http://www.cdc.gov/nip/vacsafe/vaccinesafety/sideeffects/autism.htm.)

Sharon Humiston, whose son is autistic, feels very strongly that parents should not accept it as common knowledge that vaccines cause autism. The association between autism and MMR may simply be based on the fact that MMR is given shortly before the time in a child's life when parents begin expecting them to speak. She says, "Families should demand the same level of science (and, thus, the same level of expenditures) for autism as would go into comparable epidemics."

*Q: Does MMR cause inflammatory bowel disease?*

Researchers in Sweden and the United Kingdom hypothesized this link, but other researchers have not been able replicate their work. To date, no study that is accepted by the scientific community has shown a link between MMR vaccine and inflammatory bowel syndrome. (See http://www.vaccinesafety.edu/mmrandibd.htm.)

*Q: Does MMR cause diabetes?*

No. Infection with wild mumps virus has been shown to trigger diabetes in some individuals. Mumps vaccine virus is a much weakened version of the wild virus and no association has been made between it and diabetes (or other damage to the pancreas).

*Q: Is there concern that giving measles, mumps, and rubella vaccines together is more likely to cause problems for the child than giving them separately? Or for that matter, do any combination of vaccines pose a similar problem?*

If a child gets two infections at the same time, the rate of complications is simply additive. It is the same with immunizations. Before licensure, the FDA requires studies in which vaccines are given simultaneously.

*Q: Is it true that MMR vaccine won't provide lifelong immunity? If it won't, why not just get the diseases?*

Immunity from MMR vaccine usually lasts a lifetime. Studies have shown that waning immunity is not a big problem after MMR. Furthermore, there are risks of complications from the diseases themselves.

*Q: Did rubella vaccine trigger an epidemic of Epstein-Barr syndrome?*

No. Epstein-Barr syndrome is more commonly known as infectious mononucleosis, or mono for short. Epstein-Barr is in the herpes family of viruses, which are not even remotely related to rubella virus.

*Q: Why not just vaccinate adolescent girls and women of childbearing age for immunity to rubella instead of immunizing babies?*

Some countries use that strategy to prevent congenital rubella syndrome. In the U.S., we have not been extremely successful with immunization programs after early childhood. By immunizing twice before adolescence, we ensure that all females are protected well before sexual contact.

*Q: Why would my son need rubella vaccine when that disease now poses a danger mainly for unborn children?*

Boys are immunized with this vaccine to prevent the spread of rubella, since they too develop the disease and transmit it to others.

*Q: About 10 days after receiving MMR, my child broke out in a rash. Should I have kept her home from daycare?*

Children vaccinated with MMR don't spread the vaccine viruses, not even if they develop a rash after vaccination. Your child need not stay home. Of course, you may want to keep your child out of daycare if she has a fever and feels cranky.

## WHAT DOES THE FUTURE HOLD?

MMR may be combined with chickenpox vaccine, so a single injection will prevent four diseases, but we do not know when such a vaccine will be licensed.

*Eat no green apples or you'll droop.*
*Be careful not to get the croup.*
*Avoid the chickenpox and such,*
*And don't fall out of windows much.*

—Edward Anthony

# Chapter 13

# Chickenpox (Varicella) Vaccine

Unless vaccinated, nearly everyone will become infected by chickenpox, most often in early childhood or later on when complications are more likely. In the United States before a vaccine was available, chickenpox infected 3.7 million people a year, hospitalized more than 10,000, and killed 100, about 40 of whom were children (see Figure 13-1).

Controversies surround the current recommendation to give chickenpox vaccine to all U.S. infants. A great concern is that the immunity from the vaccine may wear off years later, when the individual is much older and so has a far greater risk for complications from the disease. Also, because chickenpox is considered a relatively mild childhood disease, some parents believe that vaccination is unnecessary. Complaints have been raised that this is a "designer vaccine," meaning it was developed for parents' convenience, so they wouldn't have to miss work. Use of the vaccine is increasing, though: in 1997, 26 percent of 2 year olds were vaccinated against chickenpox, whereas just a year later, 43 percent were vaccinated. As of this writing, chickenpox vaccine requirements have been enacted in 14 states, with more on the way.

**Figure 13-1**
## INCIDENCE OF CHICKENPOX, BY AGE

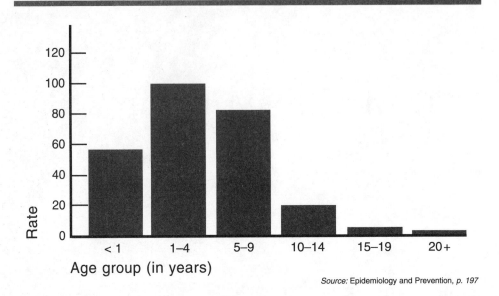

Source: Epidemiology and Prevention, p. 197

## THE CHICKENPOX DISEASE

### What is chickenpox, and how is it spread?

Chickenpox is the common name for a disease caused by the varicella virus. It is spread from person to person, via airborne droplets of mucus from the upper airway of infected people. It is also spread by direct contact with the fluid in the pox. An infected person can unknowingly spread the disease before his or her symptoms appear. Without vaccination, almost everyone gets chickenpox. If one person has it, about 85 percent of his or her susceptible close contacts will get it, too.

The illness begins with fever and malaise for a day or two, and then the rash breaks out. Crops of spots show up on the scalp and back of the neck, then on the trunk and extremities. The spots start to look like pimples and then change to blisters with a red base. Over the five or six days after the first spots appear, new ones show up and turn to blisters as the first ones crust over. Although some lucky people hardly even know they have chickenpox infection, on average people get 250 to 500 of these itchy blisters—and the more blisters, the higher the fever (see Figure 13-2).

The blisters can become infected with bacteria, causing scars or worse. In recent years, bacteria that are not killed by antibiotics have invaded chickenpox blisters and caused unstoppable tissue destruction and several gruesome deaths. Other complications of community-acquired, or wild, chickenpox are low platelet count and inflammation of the joints, kidneys, liver, brain, or the meninges.

A fetus exposed to chickenpox during the first or early second trimester occasionally may be damaged, although the risk is less than that from rubella. People with weakened immune systems who are exposed to varicella virus often develop severe and prolonged illness. Also, although children often develop only mild illness, adolescents or adults often become quite sick, even developing pneumonia.

**Figure 13-2**

**CHICKENPOX (severe case in an infant)**

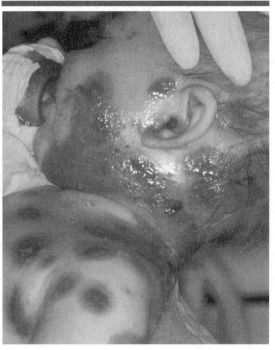

Source: American Academy of Pediatrics, Pennsylvania chapter

Shingles, a painful condition caused by the chickenpox virus, is a late-onset complication. After a person recovers from chickenpox, the virus lives on in some nerve cells. Later in life or during periods of immunosuppression (such as illness or stress), painful groups of blisters can form on the skin that these nerves serve. Because these blisters contain the virus, people can catch chickenpox from someone with shingles (but people cannot catch shingles from someone with chickenpox). About half a million persons each year suffer from shingles.

## IT HAPPENED TO GENO

Fran Friz, a mother in Los Angeles, no longer considers chickenpox just a mild childhood disease. Chickenpox nearly killed her son.

Geno was a "very healthy" 3½ year old when he came down with what became much more than an itchy childhood annoyance. Doctors said not to worry. But a few days later his fever shot up to 104 degrees and wouldn't go down, even when treated with acetaminophen. Soon Geno's skin turned "gray-green and pale in color." He wasn't eating. He slept constantly. Fran says, "no one knew what to do." So they prayed. And Fran thought she would lose her little boy.

When they returned to the doctor, Fran recalls, Geno was "pretty much unconscious." X rays showed fluid filled his lungs; one lung had shut down completely. "Had I waited a couple more hours, he would have died." Fran says that Geno developed chickenpox "inside and out," that bacteria got into "his knees and elbows," that he became "swollen from the waist down," and his "organs started shutting down."

Geno spent one month in the hospital, the first week in the intensive care unit. Fran says doctors had difficulty clearing the infection from his lungs despite the tubes put in for drainage. Doctors told Fran that during surgery they "scraped out the infection." Only then did Geno begin to feel better.

Today, as of this writing, Geno is 9 years old. But his mother continues to worry about his health. She wonders if he has a "lasting, mild learning disability" due to the disease. Fran says she wishes a chickenpox vaccine had been licensed when Geno was young so he, and the family, would not have had to endure this pain.

## THE CHICKENPOX VACCINE

### What is chickenpox vaccine, and how effective is it?

Chickenpox vaccine contains live viruses that are much like the wild chickenpox virus, but weakened. When injected under the skin of a susceptible person, the vaccine virus reproduces, causing a very mild infection. The infection is so mild that most people don't have any symptoms. The person's natural immune system develops antibodies to protect the body against future infections.

The chickenpox vaccine was licensed in the U.S. in 1995, seven years after it was licensed in Japan and Korea.

Ninety-five percent or more of healthy children and adolescents develop antibodies after vaccination. Each year after vaccination, a few percent of children will get "breakthrough disease"—that is, a mild case of chickenpox, usually fewer than 50 pox.

---

### IT HAPPENED TO ALEA

The chickenpox vaccine didn't entirely work for 6-year-old Alea. Six months after the little girl from Atlanta, Georgia, received the vaccine, she developed a mild case of the disease.

Her mother, Amy, says she was surprised. She thought Alea would have been protected. Still, she says her daughter's case of chickenpox was milder than most, probably due to the vaccine. She doesn't regret having Alea immunized for chickenpox.

---

## Who should get chickenpox vaccine and when?

**Children.** CDC and the AAP recommend chickenpox vaccine for most children 12 months to 12 years old who have had neither the vaccine nor the disease. One dose of chickenpox vaccine is given at 12 to 18 months of age. No repeat doses are recommended at this time.

**Adolescents and adults.** ACIP recommends vaccination for people who are likely to be exposed to the virus: teachers of young children and daycare employees, residents and staff in institutional settings and correctional facilities, college students, military personnel, people living in households with children, and international travelers. Vaccination is also recommended for people who have close contact with others who may get serious complications if they are exposed to the virus, such as healthcare workers and family contacts of immunosuppressed people. ACIP considers vaccination of other adolescents and adults desirable as part of routine healthcare visits.

For anyone 13 years old or older, two doses separated by at least four weeks are needed. No repeat doses beyond the initial pair are recommended at this time.

To prevent chickenpox during pregnancy, women should be sure they are immune *before* they become pregnant. Women should not receive the vaccine during pregnancy or become pregnant for one month afterward.

Also, ACIP recommends giving the vaccine to susceptible children and adults who have been exposed to the wild virus. The vaccine is 70 to 100 percent effective if used within three days of exposure. It may be effective even longer, possibly up to five days after the exposure.

## Who should *not* get the vaccine?

Chickenpox vaccine should *not* be given to anyone who has the following reactions or conditions:

- A serious allergic reaction to a prior dose of chickenpox vaccine or to a prior exposure to its contents (such as gelatin, neomycin).

- A problem with his or her immune system. People with HIV infection who don't have symptoms of AIDS may receive chickenpox vaccine. People with an immuno-compromised household member may receive chickenpox vaccine.

- Pregnancy (but chickenpox vaccine may be given to children with a pregnant household member).

- A moderate to severe illness. The vaccine should be given when the person is feeling better.

- The recent receipt of a blood product that contains antibodies (such as immune globulin). Discuss this with your healthcare provider.

## What are the vaccine risks and side effects?

In addition to allergic reactions that can occur after any vaccine, the following are some other risks and side effects that have been known to occur after chickenpox vaccine.

- Pain and/or redness at the injection site occur within the first day or two in 15 to 20 percent of children and as many as 33 percent of adolescents. About 4 percent of vaccine recipients will develop two to four pox at the injection site.

✛ Body rash—ten or fewer pox—may develop 7 to 21 days after vaccination and usually resolves within a few days. About 4 percent of susceptible people experience this.

✛ Fever may begin 7 to 12 days after vaccination and usually resolves within a day or two. About 14 percent of susceptible children and fewer adolescents experience this. Some children have seizures when they develop a fever, irrespective of the cause of the fever.

✛ Shingles, to date, is at least four to five times less common after chickenpox vaccine than after chickenpox disease. People who do get shingles after the vaccine have a mild case without complications. No one knows if these vaccine benefits will remain true over the long term.

✛ Seizure (jerking or staring), caused by fever, occurs in less than 1 person out of 1,000.

## WHAT OTHER QUESTIONS DO PARENTS ASK?

*Q: Will immunity to chickenpox wane many years after vaccination, leaving people susceptible during childbearing years or later, when the risk of serious chickenpox is higher than it is during childhood?*

Twenty years after immunization, follow-up studies in Japan show lasting immunity. In the U.S. where the vaccine has not been in use as long, follow-up studies also show that almost all vaccinated individuals remain immune.

*Q: Will the use of chickenpox vaccine by some, but not all, U.S. children cause unvaccinated children to be less likely to be exposed to chickenpox until later in life?*

Chickenpox virus spreads easily from person to person, so before the vaccine was available, most people were exposed as children. Now, with about half of all children in the U.S. receiving the vaccine, unvaccinated children are somewhat more likely to reach adolescence still susceptible to chickenpox. If exposed as teenagers, there is an increased chance of complications.

If all children were vaccinated, this would not be an issue. If your child is vaccinated, it is not an issue for your family. But if you choose not to have your infant vaccinated, when he or she reaches 11 or 12 you should discuss with the child's pediatrician getting a chickenpox vaccination or a blood test to show if your child needs the vaccine.

*Q: Can my child catch chickenpox from someone who has had the vaccine?*

A child who develops a rash after receiving the varicella vaccine can spread the weakened vaccine virus but not the wild virus. The weakened vaccine virus does not cause symptoms.

*Q: Shouldn't I wait till the vaccine has been around longer since long-term effects are still unknown?*

Data collection in the United States on the safety and efficacy of the chickenpox vaccine began several years before the vaccine was licensed in 1995 and has been ongoing since licensure. Japan has collected over 20 years of data on a very similar vaccine. If you are determined to wait, it would be wise to reconsider having your child vaccinated or tested for immunity at the age 11 or 12 doctor visit.

*Q: Should the vaccine be recommended for all infants or only for susceptible adolescents?*

From a large-scale, purely economic viewpoint, vaccinating only susceptible adolescents has the advantage over vaccinating all infants. However, if parents want their children protected as soon as possible, this strategy is not optimal.

*Q: Should immuno-compromised individuals and their susceptible close contacts get the vaccine?*

At this time, people with weakened immune systems should not get this vaccine, but the people around them should. There is concern that the live viruses in the chickenpox vaccine could cause severe disease in people whose immune systems are too weak to kill them off. For this reason, in the U.S.

chickenpox vaccine is not licensed for use in immuno-compromised people (except those with asymptomatic HIV and those with immune deficiencies limited to their antibody-making cells). Further research results may show the vaccine to be safe and effective for immuno-compromised people. Until then, it is very important for people who have close contact with immuno-compromised individuals to ensure they are immune to chickenpox.

*Q: My child is 16 now, and I don't think she had chickenpox, but I'm not sure. If she did have chickenpox and now she gets the vaccine, is that dangerous?*

No. Vaccination of people who were already immune has not led to more side effects.

*Q: A child in my child's daycare developed chickenpox rash yesterday. My child never got the vaccine. Is it too late now?*

No. Chickenpox vaccine does reduce the likelihood of getting chickenpox symptoms, especially if given within the first three days after the exposure.

*Q: After receiving chickenpox vaccine my child broke out in a rash. Should I keep her home from daycare?*

Yes. It is hard to tell at first if a child who breaks out in a rash after varicella vaccine has a side effect from the vaccine—which is unlikely to spread to other children—or if it is real chickenpox that was brewing before the vaccine was given. Most daycare sites have a "no rash" policy, so they will exclude the child until the pox crust, whatever the cause of the rash.

*Q: Is it dangerous to get the MMR vaccine at the same visit as the chickenpox vaccine?*

No. Testing has not shown any increase in side effects when these vaccines are given on the same day. ACIP, AAP, and AAFP strongly recommend giving these and other needed vaccines at the same visit.

*Q: If I opt not to get my child vaccinated for chickenpox, are there things I can do to prevent severe reaction from the disease?*

Yes. Pox should be kept clean and signs of bacterial infection (redness, pus, foul odor) should be brought to medical attention. A child with chickenpox should never be given aspirin, only acetaminophen (such as Tylenol™) or ibuprofen (such as Advil™). Children who get aspirin when they have chickenpox (or influenza) may become disoriented, combative, and stuporous as part of Reye syndrome.

*Q: Is there anything (other than the vaccine) that successfully treats chickenpox?*

Intravenous concentrated chickenpox antibodies (varicella zoster immune globulin or VZIG) are given to immuno-compromised susceptible people if they are accidentally exposed to someone with chickenpox. There are also antiviral medications that can be given. Although these are considered important therapy for immuno-compromised individuals, they are rarely used in those with a normal immune system.

## WHAT DOES THE FUTURE HOLD?

Chickenpox may be combined with MMR vaccine, so one injection will prevent four diseases, but no time frame has been proposed for it. A vaccine for shingles is being studied by the National Institutes for Health. The hope is that this vaccine would reduce the likelihood of shingles if given to adults who had wild chickenpox disease as children. This vaccine, which is many times stronger than the one given to prevent chickenpox, will not be through its tests for effectiveness until 2003 or later.

# Chapter 14

# Hepatitis A Vaccine

In the United States, Hepatitis A is one of the most commonly reported diseases that can be prevented by a vaccine. The CDC estimates that each year in the U.S. 180,000 people contract hepatitis A, half of whom develop no symptoms and therefore spread it unknowingly. Although an effective vaccine has been available here since 1995, about 100 people still die each year from liver failure caused by hepatitis A.

In North America cases of hepatitis A have peaked in 1954, 1961, and in the early 1970s. Smaller peaks were noted in the late 1980s and mid-1990s (see Figure 14-1). As sanitary conditions improve, these peaks every 5 to 10 years have involved many fewer people.

Like polio, hepatitis A is most common in children, probably because it is spread in the stool. Also like polio, hepatitis A tends to cause more severe disease in adults. Among preschool children, only about 30 percent get symptoms, but more than 70 percent of older children and adults get symptoms from hepatitis A infection. Three out of 1,000 persons who contract hepatitis A die from it, but 18 out of 1,000 people die in the 50 and older age group.

Hepatitis A vaccine has not been very controversial up to now because most of the people receiving it have been adults who suspected they would

**Figure 14-1**

## HEPATITIS A IN THE UNITED STATES, 1966–1998

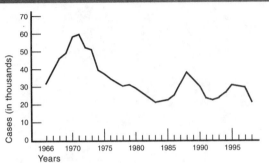

Source: *Epidemiology and Prevention, p. 213*

be exposed to hepatitis A, for example, during travel to a developing country. In 1999, CDC recommended the vaccine for all children 2 to 18 years old in states, counties, or communities where hepatitis A virus infections are common (mainly in the western states).

Parents may be concerned about giving the vaccine to their child since hepatitis A is rarely life threatening and not a significant risk until later in life. The purpose of CDC's recommendation is both to protect individuals and to stop the spread of the hepatitis A virus. Like many germs that are spread in stool, children spread the hepatitis A virus to other children, but studies in the U.S. have shown that children also often spread the disease to adults who are not already immune.

A second concern is vaccine safety. Before licensing, hepatitis A vaccines were carefully evaluated for safety. Since the vaccine was licensed, it has been administered to millions more. Now that the vaccine is recommended as a routine childhood vaccine in some areas of the country, many times the number of children who received it previously will receive it between the years 2000 and 2005. Will the vaccination of millions of children reveal previously unsuspected problems? It is very unlikely, but CDC has identified the evaluation of hepatitis A vaccine safety as an issue that should be addressed in future studies.

Finally, another potential concern is that, like chickenpox, hepatitis A tends to be a more serious disease if one's first exposure comes later in life. Unlike the vaccine against chickenpox, however, the vaccine against hepatitis A is inactivated (not live), so there is less certainty that it will provide lifelong immunity. By giving the vaccine during childhood, are we only postponing the disease until later in life when its danger increases? As of this writing, the longest currently available study is seven years, and it shows that the vaccine is continuing to protect. On the basis of current data, scientists expect the vaccine to work for 20 years or more. CDC is conducting studies to evaluate the long-term protection afforded by hepatitis A vaccine. Just as with chickenpox, children who receive the vaccine in the first decade of the twenty-first century and who live in communities with a high prevalence of hepatitis A will continue to receive boosters through exposure to the live virus out in the community.

## THE HEPATITIS A DISEASE

### What is hepatitis A, and how is it spread?

Hepatitis A is a virus that multiplies in the body for about four weeks before symptoms of liver damage begin. The infected person then develops fever, nausea, appetite loss, dark urine, and jaundice (the skin takes on a yellow cast and the whites of the eyes turn yellow). Most people have these symptoms for less than two months. But 10 to 15 percent of persons with these symptoms suffer from them continuously or on and off for up to six months.

The most common way for hepatitis A to spread is for the tiniest bit of stool from an infected person—with or without symptoms—to get in the mouth of another person. It sounds awful, but our daycare centers, our homes, and our children's hands are often not as clean as we imagine. Hepatitis A also can be spread when someone with "dirty" hands prepares food for others or when sewage leaks into a water supply. A far less common route is through donated blood. When persons who have hepatitis A in their bloodstream give blood that is to be used for clotting factors, the infected blood can pass the disease to a hemophiliac.

Among hepatitis A cases that are reported to CDC, almost half were not in contact with anyone who had hepatitis symptoms. (Infected persons who had no symptoms were probably the source of the virus in these cases.) About a quarter of them had a household member or sex partner who had symptoms, although the disease is usually spread before the symptoms occur. Another 15 percent of cases were related to hepatitis A spread in daycare. (See Figure 14-2.)

Of course, many persons never know that they were infected with hepatitis A, and even those who develop symptoms do so only after several weeks of having shed the virus.

**Figure 14-2**
## SOURCE OF HEPATITIS A INFECTION

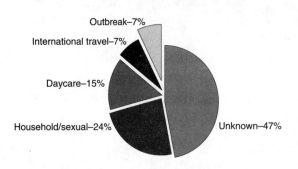

Outbreak–7%
International travel–7%
Daycare–15%
Household/sexual–24%
Unknown–47%

*Source:* Epidemiology and Prevention, *p. 212*

In nature, only humans harbor the virus. Hepatitis A virus is killed by heating food for even a minute or by washing the changing table with tap water and bleach.

### IT HAPPENED TO CHANDA

Chanda Luce will never forget her eleventh birthday. That's when she came down with hepatitis A. All of her friends were over for the party when she began feeling "flushed, peaked, and ill." Gayle Luce, her mom, thought it was "too much birthday celebration." But that evening Chanda drifted off while watching a movie and began vomiting during her sleep. Still, soon she was back in class.

After a few days, though, Gayle noticed that "Chanda's eyes looked yellow." After tests, doctors concluded Chanda had mononucleosis, Gayle recalls. But then the health department called, saying "they thought she had hepatitis A." Chanda's entire class of 27 kids, all of those at the birthday party, plus additional family and friends (about 50 people in all) had to be vaccinated. Chanda's parents had to track down everyone she had come into contact with. "Even her teacher had to get a shot." Some of the boys at school "were going to a ballgame but had to stop at the health department for shots first." Chanda missed more than a week of school and weeks of horseback riding and softball games.

Gayle Luce explains that they never found out exactly how her daughter contracted hepatitis A. They had not been traveling in some exotic third world country where the disease is common. Since it occurred shortly after their school in Olympia, Washington, instituted cafeteria style lunches, she suspects a sick child may have touched the food, contaminating it with fecal matter, passing on the disease.

Gayle says, "It was one of the worst things I've ever gone through." She missed work to care for her daughter, she watched her usually energetic child feel sick and exhausted, and Gayle was embarrassed. She says Chanda is meticulous and from a clean household. She wonders how she could have gotten hepatitis. "Oh, yuck," she said. "If you get it, something is wrong. I didn't want to make her feel bad, but every time she went to the bathroom I had to disinfect everything."

Gayle's advice: "I wish she had not had to go through it. I would recommend other people get the vaccine, especially if you are traveling. It's not fun."

## What are the risk factors for hepatitis A disease?

**Age.** By checking the blood for evidence of hepatitis A, researchers have found that while only 9 percent of U.S. children aged 6 to 11 have ever been infected with hepatitis A, 75 percent of those older than 70 have been previously infected. The disease is more of a threat to people infected at an older age.

**Race/ethnicity and poverty.** Persons who are poor are more likely to become infected with hepatitis A. In the U.S., the highest rates are among Native Americans and Alaskan Natives. Contact with people from countries where hepatitis A is endemic (such as Mexico, Central and South America) also increases the risk of exposure to the disease. When adjustments are made for age, Mexican Americans are more likely to show evidence of having had hepatitis A (70 percent), then blacks (39 percent) and whites (23 percent).

**Region.** In the U.S., hepatitis A is most common in the western states (see Figure 14-3). Half of all reported cases come from 11 states with only 22 percent of the U.S. population. These states include

| | |
|---|---|
| Arizona | Washington |
| Alaska | Oklahoma |
| Oregon | South Dakota |
| New Mexico | Nevada |
| Utah | California |
| Idaho | |

Six more states also have a bit more than their share of hepatitis A. These states, with 12 percent of the population, have 16 percent of the hepatitis A:

| | |
|---|---|
| Missouri | Arkansas |
| Texas | Montana |
| Colorado | Wyoming |

**Other risk factors.** The following persons are at increased risk of contracting hepatitis A:

✛ Travelers to developing countries. Worldwide, hepatitis A is less common in developed countries (such as Scandinavia, parts of western Europe, North America, Japan, Australia, and New Zealand) than in the developing world (see Figure 14-4). In the developing world, however, outbreaks are uncommon because most people become immune after they are exposed in early childhood. Travelers from developed to developing countries are at notable risk. If leaving in less than four weeks, instead of the vaccine, travelers can opt for a concentrate of hepatitis A antibodies (called immune globulin), which gives three months of protection. The combination of the vaccine and immune globulin gives more complete and more lasting protection than the immune globulin alone.

✛ Sexually active male homosexuals

✛ Illegal-drug users

✛ People who work with hepatitis A virus or hepatitis A–infected primates in a research setting

✛ People who take clotting-factor concentrates, especially those treated with solvents or detergents

During an outbreak of hepatitis A, local public health authorities should be consulted to decide if vaccination is needed.

**Figure 14-3**

## AREAS WHERE HEPATITIS A WAS MOST PREVALENT, THROUGH 1997

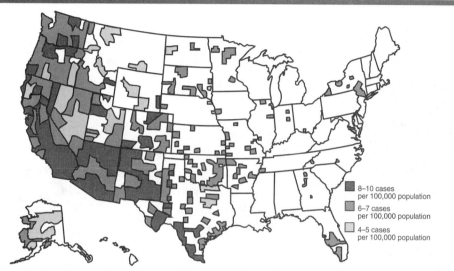

- 8–10 cases per 100,000 population
- 6–7 cases per 100,000 population
- 4–5 cases per 100,000 population

*Source: National Notifiable Disease Surveillance System; MMWR 48, RR-12, 1999, p.7*

**Figure 14-4**

## HEPATITIS A INFECTION WORLDWIDE

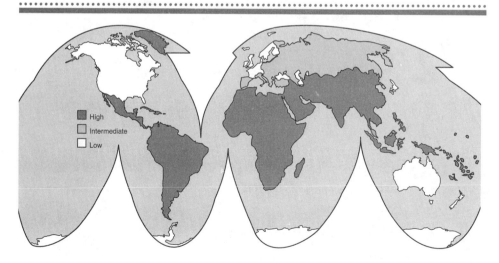

- High
- Intermediate
- Low

*Source: MMWR 48, RR-12, 1999, p.11*

# The Hepatitis A Vaccine

### What is the hepatitis A vaccine, and how effective is it?

Like the inactivated polio vaccine (IPV), hepatitis A vaccine contains whole viruses that have been killed (or "inactivated") by formalin. Almost all people who received the recomended two doses of either brand of hepatitis A vaccine have been protected by it. This is a remarkably effective vaccine, rivaling the live vaccines.

### Who should get the hepatitis A vaccine and when?

Currently, this vaccine is only licensed for people who are 2 years of age or older. Infants should not receive hepatitis A vaccine. Two doses of the vaccine are recommended for all ages. The second dose should be given no sooner than six months after the first.

ACIP recommends hepatitis A vaccination for people who have chronic liver disease (because they may have severe consequences if infected) and for people who have a higher than average risk of being infected. The latter group includes those persons in groups detailed above as well as all children in certain communities, specifically

- ✛ Children living in areas where the incidence is highest (including the 11 states listed above). ACIP recommends that these children should be vaccinated. Emphasis should be on children beginning at age 2 years, with catch-up at preschool, and, if feasible, inclusion of all children up to 15 years of age.

- ✛ Children living in areas where the incidence is intermediate (including the six states listed above). ACIP says that in these places hepatitis A vaccine *should be considered* for routine use. Emphasis in these areas should be on children in a particular age group (such as those entering middle school), a particular setting (such as daycare), or a setting convenient for immunization (such as when seeking healthcare for other reasons).

## Who should *not* get the vaccine?

Hepatitis A vaccine should not be given to your child if he or she

✛ Is less than 2 years old.

✛ Had a serious allergic reaction to a prior dose of hepatitis A vaccine.

✛ Has a moderate to severe illness. If this is the case, the child may receive the vaccine when feeling better.

## What are the vaccine risks and side effects?

Allergic reactions could occur after any vaccine. These are the other risks and side effects that have been known to occur after hepatitis A vaccines:

✛ Minor pain or tenderness, swelling, or warmth at the injection site may begin soon after the shot and usually resolve within a day. Between 15 and 19 percent of children will experience pain or tenderness; fewer experience warmth (9 percent). Among adults, more than half report some pain or tenderness at the injection site.

✛ General side effects may include headache (4 percent of children, 14 percent of adults), "just not feeling well" (7 percent of adults), or poor feeding (8 percent of children).

✛ Serious side effects appear to be uncommon. After millions of people around the world have taken the vaccine, no serious side effect has been attributed to hepatitis A vaccine.

## WHAT OTHER QUESTIONS DO PARENTS ASK?

*Q: Isn't it better for my child to contract hepatitis A as a child when the disease will be milder and give him lifelong immunity?*

Although children may have mild illness, serious illness and complications may occur in this age group. In addition, children with hepatitis A may transmit the infection to older people who are at increased risk of more severe illness and complications.

Q: *What if my child got the first dose of the vaccine a couple of years ago? Do we have to start over?*

No, there is no need to start over from the beginning. After six months, a second dose is recommended as soon as feasible, though.

Q: *There are two brands of vaccine. Do we need to have the same brand for both doses?*

No, it isn't necessary to get the same brand both times.

Q: *I'm going to Cairo, Egypt, so I may be exposed to hepatitis A while on the trip. But I'm 40, so it's likely that I have already been exposed. Should I get the vaccine or not?*

You should discuss these two options with your healthcare provider: you can (1) get the vaccine—if it turns out that you already had the infection, then there's no harm done—or (2) get a blood test to see if you are already immune. The drawback is that if it turns out that you are not already immune, you have to get back in for the vaccine at least four weeks before your departure. Also, the cost of the test may be more than the cost of the vaccine, so that's another consideration to discuss.

Q: *My family is leaving for Mexico in a couple of weeks. We'll only be on vacation for a week. Should we bother with the vaccine now?*

If you are traveling in less than four weeks to a country where hepatitis A is common, such as Mexico, you should receive two injections: the hepatitis A vaccine, plus a concentrate of hepatitis A antibodies (called hepatitis A immune globulin). Although many people develop their own antibodies even two weeks after vaccination, it's best not to bet on it. Also, if you want long-term protection, you will need a second dose of the vaccine at least six months after the first dose.

## WHAT DOES THE FUTURE HOLD?

It's likely that a growing number of states will recommend that children be vaccinated for hepatitis A. Also, a hepatitis A–hepatitis B vaccine combination might be available in the U.S. in the first decade of the twenty-first century. But, like all vaccines in development, there is no guarantee when or if it will make it through the FDA licensing process.

Chapter 15

# Pneumococcal Vaccine

Most parents have heard of strep throat, but one family of strep, *Streptococcus pneumoniae,* or pneumococcus, deserves special attention. Pneumococcal disease is the most common cause of vaccine-preventable death in the United States, killing more people than all other vaccine-preventable diseases combined. These bacteria present significant danger for both the youngest and oldest members of our families. The disease is now the most common cause of bacterial meningitis in babies. One quarter of cases occur in children under age 5, resulting in 17,000 cases of serious invasive pneumococcal disease every year in children in this age group. In children under age 5, annually in the U.S., pneumococcus causes

- 16,300 cases of bloodstream infections,

- 700 cases of bacterial meningitis,

- 5 million ear infections, and

- 200 deaths.

For people of all ages each year in the U.S., pneumococcus causes

- 500,000 cases of pneumococcal pneumonia,

✚ 60,000 cases of bacteremia (that is, bacteria in the bloodstream that can lead to high fevers, pneumonia, or meningitis),

✚ 3,000 cases of meningitis, and

✚ up to 11,000 deaths.

In the 1880s, scientists first began to understand pneumococcus. In the 1940s, shortly after penicillin proved to be successful in treating certain bacterial infections, a study showed that a pneumococcal vaccine could prevent some infections in military recruits. By 1977, a vaccine was licensed that contained 14 different strains of pneumococcus, and in 1983 a 23-strain vaccine was licensed, but only for children older than 2 and for adults.

Unfortunately, children younger than 2 years bear much of the burden of pneumococcal disease. The incidence of invasive pneumococcal disease is 165 per 100,000 for children up to 12 months, 203 cases per 100,000 for children aged 12 to 23 months, with the peak occurring among children aged 6 to 11 months (at 235 per 100,000). Incidence of the disease among adults aged 65 and older is 61 per 100,000. In contrast, incidence among persons of all ages is 24 per 100,000. (see Figure 15-1).

A hundred years after pneumococcus was first isolated and shown to be a major cause of pneumonia, development began on a vaccine that could prevent pneumococcal disease in infants and young children. The vaccine was recommended by ACIP in October 1999 even before it was licensed by the FDA.

**Figure 15-1**
## INCIDENCE OF PNEUMOCOCCAL DISEASE, BY AGE, 1998

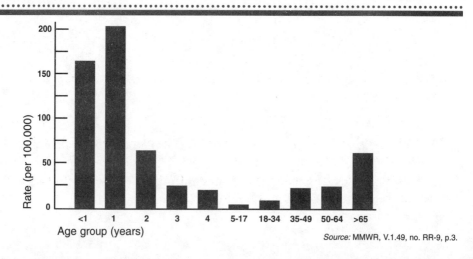

*Source:* MMWR, V.1.49, no. RR-9, p.3.

## THE PNEUMOCOCCAL DISEASE

### What is pneumococcal disease, and how is it spread?

There are at least 90 different strains of the bacteria pneumococcus, or *Streptococcus pneumoniae*. Though most pneumococcal strains can cause serious disease in humans, 10 strains are estimated to cause more than 60 percent of invasive disease worldwide. Certain strains have tended to dominate in different places, during different times in history, and in different age groups. Currently in the U.S., seven strains account for about 80 percent of invasive pneumococcal infections in children younger than 6 years old.

The bacteria live in the mucus of the nose and throat of many people who don't get ill from it. The bacteria spread when the person carrying them sprays droplets by coughing or sneezing. Another person picks up the disease by inhaling the infected airborne droplets. Most commonly, pneumococcus causes 30 to 60 percent or more of all middle-ear infections. Ninety-one percent of children have at least one middle-ear infection before they're 2 years old. This kind of infection can have significant consequences, such as hearing impairment, delayed language development, and cognitive problems. The financial costs also can be significant: *$3.5 billion* each year for medical expenses and lost work time.

Although *viruses* are the most frequent cause of pneumonia in children, pneumococcus is the most frequent *bacterial* cause of pneumonia among older children who need to be hospitalized. An estimated 135,000 children are hospitalized each year in the U.S. for pneumococcal pneumonia. Similarly, among adults, pneumococcal infections are the major cause of pneumonia that requires hospitalization.

In the U.S., pneumococcus is the most common cause of bacterial meningitis among children younger than 5 years and the cause of 13 to 19 percent of all bacterial meningitis. About 20 percent of patients with pneumococcal meningitis die from it, and among those who survive, 25 to 30 percent have serious nervous system aftereffects such as mental retardation, a long-term seizure disorder, or hearing loss.

Many antibiotics are available to treat the various strains of pneumococcal disease. Unfortunately, more and more of these strains are becoming resistant to antibiotics. Newer antibiotics are being developed to keep ahead of the problem, but the best way to attack pneumococcus is to prevent the infection in the first place by vaccinating.

## Who gets pneumococcal disease?

For a person to become ill from the disease, the pneumococcal bacteria have to spread from his or her nose or throat to the bloodstream, which then carries the germs to the lungs or brain. The risk of contracting the disease probably is higher among children younger than 6 because they have not yet developed immunity to pneumococci and because their immune systems are not mature.

Adults are at risk of contracting the disease if their immune systems are weakened by HIV infection or cancer, chemotherapy or prolonged courses of high-dose prednisone, kidney or liver disease, a damaged spleen, diabetes, or alcoholism. Among adults with a healthy immune system, the risk of invasive disease increases if, for example, they can't clear the mucus in their airways because the cells have been poisoned by cigarette smoke or other air pollutants or if their cough and gag reflexes have been dulled by old age, alcohol, or drugs.

---

### IT HAPPENED TO JACOB

Carla Newby shared her tragic story with those listening at an Advisory Committee on Immunization Practices meeting in October 1999. She talked about her son Jacob, a first grader, "an all-American kid—no special medical problems," who had to be hospitalized for what turned out to be pneumococcal meningitis. Carla explained he "was in a hospital dying, ... but they did not act quickly enough to diagnose Jacob's meningitis, and start the proper treatment." She said, "The result was tragic." Her son, not quite 7 years old, died from pneumococcal meningitis in late October 1998.

Carla noted that Jacob's case isn't unusual. Serving as general manager of the Meningitis Foundation of America, she speaks with parents across the country every day whose children are misdiagnosed or "at best diagnosed very late, causing delays in treatment."

Jacob, Carla pointed out, had none of the conditions that would have prompted his doctor to give him the pneumococcal vaccine which used to be recommended only for children in high-risk groups. "But he still got pneumococcal meningitis."

Carla Newby lamented, "The hardest thing I have ever had to do was tell my baby that it was okay to stop fighting and let go."

---

## THE PNEUMOCOCCAL VACCINE

### What is the pneumococcal vaccine, and how effective is it?

The pneumococcal vaccines are of two types, neither of which contains live bacteria. The newly licensed vaccine (PCV7, or pneumococcal conjugate vaccine) is effective against the seven types of pneumococcus that most frequently cause disease in infants and young children. The vaccine works in infants and young children, produces higher antibody levels with each dose, and produces a long-lasting immune response.

In a prelicensure study of almost 38,000 healthy children who received four doses of PCV7, the vaccine proved to be 97 percent effective in preventing pneumococcus from infecting the blood or spinal fluid. Many germs cause pneumonia, so PCV7 would not be expected to prevent all pediatric pneumonia, but in the same trial the new vaccine reduced by 33 percent the number of cases of pneumonia severe enough to show up on an X ray. Similarly, ear infections are caused by many germs, and the vaccine does not prevent all of them, but it does reduce by more than 20 percent the number of children with frequent ear infections.

The other pneumococcal vaccine (PPV23, or pure polysaccharide vaccine), which has been in use since 1983 for children age 2 and older and for adults, is effective against the 23 types of pneumococcus that cause at least 90 percent of all pneumococcal disease in the U.S. Various studies have shown PPV23 to be 56 to 81 percent effective in preventing invasive pneumococcal disease, but it may not be as effective in persons with weakened immune systems. It also is not effective against ear infections caused by pneumococcus.

### Who should get the vaccine and when?

**Young children.** PCV7 is routinely recommended for all children 6 weeks to 23 months of age. Also, the vaccine is recommended for children 24 to 59 months of age who are at very high risk for pneumococcal disease—that is, those who have a long-term health problem including heart disease, diabetes, lung disease (other than asthma), sickle-cell disease, liver disease, or an open direct path between the nose and the brain (that is, a "CSF leak"). Children also are at risk for pneumococcal disease if they have a weakened immune system due to cancer or cancer treatment, damaged or no spleen, long-term steroids, kidney disease, HIV or AIDS, or bone marrow or organ transplant. Other children who are most likely to benefit from the new vaccine are children who have frequent ear infections, attend group childcare, live in poverty, or are Alaskan Natives, a member of certain Native American populations, or African American.

The number of doses recommended depends on when a child starts the series and if he or she is at risk for pneumococcal disease. Here is a summary:

| Age at first dose | Number of doses recommended |
| --- | --- |
| Younger than 7 months | 3 doses plus a booster |
| 7 to 11 months | 2 doses plus a booster |
| 12 to 23 months | 2 doses (no booster) |
| Older than 23 months | |
|     Healthy | 1 dose (no booster) |
|     At high risk | 2 doses (no booster) |

Children who have a long-term health problem or a weakened immune system and who completed the series of PCV7 before 2 years of age should receive one dose of the old pneumococcal vaccine, PPV23. This should be received at the age of 2, at least eight weeks after receiving the final PCV7.

**Older children and adults.** The original pneumococcal vaccine, PPV23, is recommended for all people 65 and older, even if they are healthy. It is also recommended for persons 6 and older if they are at high risk for pneumococcal disease. The factors that increase an older child's or adult's risk of pneumococcal disease are the same as for young children, specifically a long-term health problem (including alcoholism), a weakened immune system, or being an Alaskan Native or a member of certain Native American populations.

Only one dose of PPV23 is recommended for most of these persons. A second dose is recommended for those who have a long-term health problem or weakened immune system.

## Who should *not* get the vaccine?

Neither pneumococcal vaccine should be given to a person if he or she had a serious allergic reaction to a prior dose of pneumococcal vaccine or has a moderate to severe illness. If the latter is the case, the person may receive the vaccine when feeling better.

## What are the vaccine risks and side effects?

Allergic reactions could occur after any vaccine, but they are rare. For PCV7, the new vaccine for infants, the side effects are as follows:

✚ Mild pain or tenderness, swelling, or warmth at the injection site occur in more than 33 percent of the children after each vaccine dose.

✚ A low-grade fever occurs in 22 to 38 percent of children after each vaccine dose, though it is not known how many of these fevers were caused by the other routine vaccines (such as DTP) that were given at the same time. Since DTaP is now recommended for children, the incidence of fevers should diminish.

✚ Seizures due to fever also occurred in a few children who received PCV7 with DTP, but again the new DTaP should reduce these events.

✚ Deaths. A complete analysis of deaths following vaccination was not available at the time of this printing, but in the large study in Northern California, the number of deaths were evenly distributed between children who received PCV7 and those who received an experimental (meningococcus) vaccine.

No serious side effects are known to be caused by PPV23, the original vaccine. Milder side effects are as follows:

✚ Pain or tenderness, swelling, or warmth at the injection site may occur in as many as half of young adults who receive the vaccine. These side effects last one to three days. Youngsters and seniors have less of a reaction.

✚ Rash, joint or muscle pain, lymph node swelling, and fever are rare.

## WHAT OTHER QUESTIONS DO PARENTS ASK?

*Q: My mom is 73 and completely healthy. She gets the flu shot every year, but her doctor has never recommended the pneumococcal vaccine. Why not?*

This is a common oversight by physicians. Although the vaccine is recommended for all people 65 years of age and older, less than half of them get it.

*Q: My 6-year-old son still gets ear infections. Should he get the new pneumococcal vaccine?*

No. The new vaccine is not recommended for anyone older than 5 years of age.

*Q: Is it possible for other types of pneumococcus not covered by the vaccine to replace the ones that now cause disease in young children? Years from now, will there still be just as much meningitis and pneumonia as there is now?*

This is possible, but it seems unlikely from our experience with other bacterial vaccines, particularly Hib. When a large proportion of the population is using the vaccine, the health authorities will need to continue to monitor the disease rates.

## WHAT DOES THE FUTURE HOLD?

Will the use of the two pneumococcal vaccines actually decrease the amount of serious pneumococcal disease in the age groups for which they are recommended? Disease incidence must be monitored before we will know. Scientists also will be trying to find new methods for determining the effectiveness of pneumococcal vaccine and to devise optimal vaccination schedules. CDC and the FDA will scrutinize the safety of the new vaccine. Meanwhile, new technologies are being used to develop radically different and more effective pneumococcal vaccines. Eventually, our families may benefit from a pneumococcal vaccine that is delivered as a nasal spray or a liquid that can be given by mouth.

# PART THREE

---

## What You Should Know about Other Vaccines

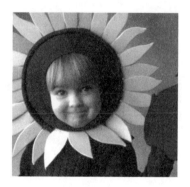

*A wise man should consider that health is the greatest*
*of human blessings.*

—Democritus

# Chapter 16

# Flu Vaccine

Today influenza, or flu, remains the second most frequent cause of death from vaccine-preventable disease in the United States. Epidemics of this highly infectious, acute viral illness were reported as early as 1510. The Spanish flu swept the world in 1918 and 1919, killing more than 20 million people, 500,000 of them in the U.S. alone. Unlike the flu today, the Spanish flu mainly killed young adults. This disease single-handedly decreased life expectancy by 10 years.

It is not surprising, then, that the tension was palpable at the CDC in the United States when, in the winter of 1997, a new and deadly strain of flu emerged in Asia. In August 1997, a young boy in Hong Kong died of a strain of flu that previously had infected only birds. By December, 17 people had been identified with the same strain of flu, and six of them had died. Epidemiologists feared that if this new flu were to spread, not just from bird to human, but from human to human, a massive pandemic could follow. Attempts to produce a vaccine failed; the viruses killed the very cells in which scientists tried to grow them. Finally, not sure if the intervention would work, officials in Hong Kong ordered the slaughter and disposal of

1.5 million chickens. No cases of this strain of flu have been identified since then, but there are no guarantees that it will not re-emerge.

The drama of pandemics should not lead us to underestimate the common flu's destructive power during a typical year. The CDC estimates that, each year on average, the flu causes 110,000 hospitalizations and 20,000 deaths in the U.S. Almost all the deaths are among the elderly and among those persons who have medical conditions, ranging from pregnancy to chronic lung disease, that predispose them to flu-related complications.

We are vulnerable to the flu each year because the virus mutates enough to get past the antibodies that our bodies formed against earlier years' strains.

## THE FLU (INFLUENZA) DISEASE

### What is flu, and how is it spread?

Influenza is a family of viruses. Influenza A and B are the two types that cause epidemics in humans.

A simple case of the flu starts suddenly, causing fever, headache, muscle aches, and exhaustion, as well as respiratory tract symptoms such as sore throat, runny or stuffy nose, and dry cough. Very young children might also experience nausea and vomiting, but these symptoms are uncommon in adults with true influenza. (The term "stomach flu" is a misnomer; other viruses and bacteria cause nausea and diarrhea in adults.) Flu infection usually is short-lived, averaging two to three days, but in some cases it can hang on for weeks, especially among the elderly.

Pneumonia is the chief complication of flu. Bacteria, which take advantage of the person's weakened state, usually cause the pneumonia. In rare circumstances, the flu virus itself will cause the pneumonia. Inflammation of the heart muscle (myocarditis), Reye syndrome, and worsening of chronic bronchitis are all infrequent complications of flu.

Flu is spread when tiny drops of mucus from the respiratory tract (the nose, throat, trachea, and lungs) of an infected person get into the respiratory tract of a susceptible person (see Figure 16-1). The droplets containing flu may be sprayed from a sneeze or cough, then inhaled or ingested on food

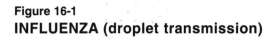

**Figure 16-1**
**INFLUENZA (droplet transmission)**

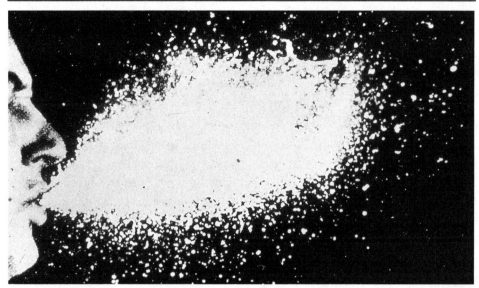

*Source: CDC*

where the droplets have landed. It can also spread from hand to mouth, via a doorknob or other inanimate object that has been handled by a person who has the flu.

Because flu passes from person to person, it spreads easily during seasons when people stay indoors, such as winter in northern climates and rainy season in the tropics.

## Who gets flu?

Although 90 percent of flu-related deaths occur in the elderly, school-aged children (age 5 to 14 years old) are infected most often and may be the major source of infection for older people. For children, flu is a major cause of fevers and ear infections, and missed school.

Flu viruses will never be eradicated. We become susceptible again each time they change. Pandemics of the flu will probably be a threat as long as there are humans to serve as virus incubators and launch pads.

### What is the best treatment for flu?

Acetaminophen (such as Tylenol™) or ibuprofen (such as Advil™) may be used to help with the fever and pain, but they do not shorten the course of the disease. In the United States, some prescription medicines, including a nasal spray, are approved for preventing or treating influenza. Though they may prevent symptoms and shorten the course of the illness by a day or two, they allow infection, so the recipient develops immunity to that flu strain. But these prescription medicines are not panaceas. Their use may cause side effects, and they are not licensed for use in children younger than 1 year old. Some strains of influenza have already mutated enough to be resistant to one of these antivirus drugs, and more resistant strains may develop. Also, these drugs do not prevent infected people from spreading the virus to others.

## THE FLU VACCINE

### What is the flu vaccine, and how effective is it?

The flu vaccine contains parts of three killed viruses: two are influenza A strains, and one is an influenza B strain. The exact strains used in the U.S. vaccine vary from year to year, depending on a scientific prediction of what flu viruses will circulate in the U.S. the following winter. This prediction is based on careful monitoring of circulating strains in Asia.

Asia is often the first place for these sitings because new strains of influenza virus originate in fowl and pigs, and many Asians live in close contact with these animals. After the new strain passes from animal to human, it then spreads around the globe from person to person.

The effectiveness of flu vaccine depends both on how accurately scientists predict which flu virus will circulate in the U.S. and on the age of the recipient. If there is a poor match between the flu viruses chosen for the vaccine and those that actually wend their way through America, the vaccine will not be very effective. Fortunately, the flu experts have usually been successful in predicting which strain will come each year.

If there is a good match, the vaccine prevents influenza in 70 to 90 percent of healthy people younger than 65, but only in 30 to 40 percent of seniors living in nursing homes. For the elderly, the real value of flu vaccine is that it helps prevent pneumonia and hospitalization (50 to 60 percent effective) and death (80 percent effective). Unvaccinated nursing home residents are twice as likely to be hospitalized and more than four times as likely to die from flu than vaccinated nursing home residents. (See Figure 16-2.)

Immunity from the vaccine wanes after vaccination and may fall below the protective level within a year, or even within a few months in the elderly. Also the virus may drift midseason, making the vaccine less effective within one flu season, and the predominant virus usually changes from year to year, so annual revaccination is necessary for protection.

## Who should get the vaccine and when?

The first year a child younger than age 9 receives flu vaccine, he or she should get two doses; the first dose is only a primer. All other eligible people should receive one dose per year. After the first year, flu vaccination should become an annual event, preferably in the early autumn months (September to mid-November).

**Figure 16-2**
## INFLUENZA COMPLICATIONS AMONG NURSING HOME RESIDENTS

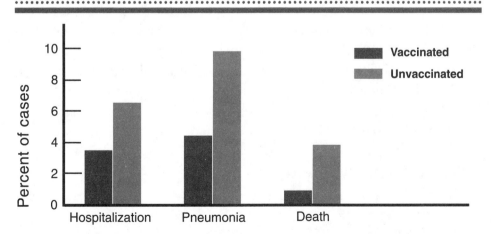

*Source:* Epidemiology and Prevention, *p. 254*

ACIP recommends that the following persons should receive the annual flu vaccine:

**People who are at high risk for flu-related complications.**

✛ Children who are 6 months to 18 years old and receive long-term aspirin therapy (a child who gets flu while taking aspirin therapy may get Reye syndrome)

✛ Children and adults who have a long-term disorder of the heart or lungs, including asthma

✛ Children and adults who have needed medical attention in the past year for a weakened immune system, kidney problems, red blood cell disorders (such as sickle-cell anemia), or a metabolic disease (such as diabetes)

✛ Women who will be in the second or third trimester of pregnancy during flu season

✛ Residents of nursing homes and other facilities who have chronic medical conditions

✛ Adults who are 50 or older (even if robustly healthy)

**People who can spread flu to those at high risk.** To protect persons at high risk of complications, ACIP recommends flu vaccine for people who live or work with the vulnerable people listed above, except pregnant women. This includes, for example, household members, caregivers, and healthcare personnel.

**Others who want to avoid flu.** Any person older than 6 months who wants to avoid the flu should get the vaccine.

## Who should *not* get the vaccine?

Flu vaccine should not be given to a person if he or she

✛ Is less than 6 months old.

✛ Had a serious allergic reaction to a prior dose of flu vaccine or hen eggs.

✛ Has a moderate to severe illness. If this is the case, the person may receive the vaccine when feeling better.

### What are the vaccine risks and side effects?

Allergic reactions could occur after any vaccine. These are the other risks and side effects that have been known to occur after flu vaccines.

✛ Minor pain or tenderness, swelling, or warmth at the injection site may begin soon after the shot and usually resolve within two days. Between 10 and 64 percent of people will experience these mild reactions.

✛ General side effects, including fever, muscle aches, or malaise may begin 6 to 12 hours after the shot and can persist for a day or two. More children than adults experience these symptoms. Overall, less than 1 percent of vaccine recipients report these side effects.

✛ Guillain-Barré syndrome, also known as GBS, causes muscle paralysis that can be severe. GBS affects 10 to 20 adults out of a million. In 1976, the swine flu vaccine caused some additional cases of GBS. Since then, it has been hard to detect any increase in GBS caused by the flu vaccine. According to the CDC, "If influenza vaccine does pose a risk [of GBS], it is probably quite small—slightly more than one additional case per million persons vaccinated."

## WHAT OTHER QUESTIONS DO PEOPLE ASK?

*Q: Can the flu vaccine cause the flu?*
No. There are no live viruses in the current flu vaccine, so they cannot replicate and start an infection. But in fewer than 1 percent of recipients the

vaccine causes fever and muscle aches. Because the vaccine does not work for about two weeks after it is given, you can get the flu if you were already infected when you received the vaccine. Also, a lot of other viruses prompt flu-like symptoms, and the vaccine does not protect you from those viruses.

*Q: Should pregnant women receive the flu vaccine, even though it has thimerosal in it?*

Thimerosal, a preservative that is about half mercury, is used in minute amounts in the flu vaccine. Experts believe that related mercury compounds should be avoided in pregnancy, but no clear-cut data are available on thimerosal. The ACIP has recommended that women who will be in their second or third trimester during flu season receive the vaccine because of their risk of serious complications from flu, but there is no such recommendation for women in their first trimester of pregnancy.

*Q: If the flu is not life threatening, isn't it better to risk getting the disease?*

Currently, the vaccine is recommended for people who are at risk for flu-related complications and for people who could spread the disease to these vulnerable persons. The other reason to get the vaccine is simply not wanting to catch flu because the disease, even in young people, can be protracted.

## WHAT DOES THE FUTURE HOLD?

A flu vaccine in the form of a nasal spray is being used in Russia and is being tested in the U.S. The potential advantages of such a vaccine are great. No needle is used, the side effects would be minimal because there would be no pain at the injection site, and immunity would develop in the lining of the nose as well as systemically.

In a preliminary study of children age 1 to 6, the intranasal flu vaccine was 93 percent effective at preventing flu and 98 percent effective against ear infections. Even parents who may not be interested in the vaccine for their healthy child who has only minimal contact with elderly persons may be relieved to have available a vaccine that prevents ear infections and other fever-related illnesses.

When the spray vaccine is licensed in the U.S., it may well be recommended for all children, not just those with medical conditions that put the children at high risk. A general recommendation would make it more likely that children with medical risks will get the vaccine and would protect the elderly as well as people with medical conditions who come in contact with children. General use of the vaccine probably would also decrease some families' medical bills and the number of days that children have to miss school and parents have to miss work.

*When you have to make a choice and don't make it,*
*that in itself is a choice.*

—William James

# Chapter 17

# Meningococcal Vaccine

Between 2,400 and 3,000 persons in the U.S. get meningococcal disease each year. About half develop meningitis, and the rest contract other systemic forms of this infection. Among people of all ages in the U.S., this comes to an annual rate of about 1 per 100,000—which is relatively low compared to, for example, the overall pneumococcal disease rate of 23 per 100,000. However, meningococcal disease warrants our attention because its effects are so severe.

## THE MENINGOCOCCAL DISEASE

### What is meningococcal disease, and how is it spread?

Meningococcus *(Neisseria meningitidis)* causes two main forms of life-threatening disease: meningitis (infection of the brain's outer lining) and meningococcemia (infection that spreads through the bloodstream). Among survivors, 10 to 19 percent will have permanent aftereffects such as deafness, mental retardation, or loss of limbs.

Meningococcus is found in the nose or throat of 5 to 11 percent of adults. The bacteria got there when an infected person sneezed or coughed, or shared another person's glass or a kiss. The bacteria penetrate the lining of the nose or throat to cause disease.

Two other groups of bacteria also have been common causes of meningitis: Hib (*Haemophilus influenzae* type b) and pneumococcus (*Streptococcus pneumoniae*). Though vaccinations during infancy can prevent Hib and pneumococcus, the current meningococcal vaccine is not very effective before age 2, which is unfortunate because the disease is most common in this younger age group.

## Who gets the disease?

Infants 3 to 12 months of age are most likely to contract meningococcal disease (see Figure 17-1). Persons have a greater risk if they have medical conditions (such as an absent or nonfunctional spleen, or HIV infection) that make it difficult to fight off the bacteria. Other risk factors for meningococcal disease include, for example, active and passive smoking, recent respiratory illness, a new residence or school, and household crowding. During outbreaks, bar or nightclub patronage and alcohol use also increase a person's risk.

Young adults are at somewhat increased risk for meningococcus. Military recruits had high rates of meningococcal disease until 1971 when they began to receive the vaccine.

**Figure 17-1**

# MENINGOCOCCAL DISEASE, BY AGE GROUP, 1989–1991

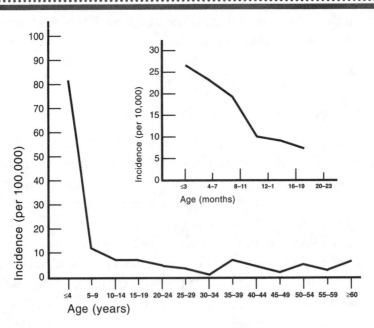

*Source: MMWR 47: RR-5, 1997*

Recent data from Maryland showed that, while most college students were at no greater risk for meningococcal disease than the general public, college students living in dormitories had a three times greater and freshmen living in dormitories had a five times greater rate of this disease than other 18 to 23 year olds. For this reason, in October 1999, ACIP recommended that college students, especially freshmen, should be made aware of meningococcal disease and the vaccine.

## How is it treated?

Antibiotics are available to treat meningococcal disease. Although the fatality rate has dropped from 70 percent in the pre-antibiotic era, 7 to 19 percent of persons with meningococcal infections still die despite proper treatment.

### IT HAPPENED TO EVAN

At the ACIP meeting in October 1999, when the meningococcal vaccine was being discussed, a mother stood up and made the following plea:

"As many of you may know, my son Evan [a college student] died from bacterial meningitis April 20, 1998. That's exactly 18 months ago today. He had been hospitalized for 26 days. Both arms and legs were amputated, and he suffered multiple organ failure.

"I'll never forget the phone call I received the morning of March 26. 'Your son has bacterial meningitis. He's in extremely critical condition. You need to get down here as soon as possible.' At that point, all I knew about meningitis was that it happened to someone else, and that it was deadly.

"It was only after Evan died that my family learned a vaccine was available that would have saved my son's life. Evan had contracted one of the serogroups that was covered by the vaccine. Then we learned that the vaccine was not something newly developed. It had been around a long time, very successfully used by the military to control outbreaks.

"The most obvious question was *why. Why* didn't we know about the vaccine? *Why* hadn't doctors told us about it? *Why* hadn't his university recommended the vaccine? *Why* was the choice to protect our son not given to us?

"We know that if we had been advised about the vaccine, our son would have received it. It wouldn't have mattered if the vaccine didn't protect against all of the serotypes, or if the vaccine didn't offer long-term immunity. What it offered was enough. Enough that Evan would have received the vaccine.

"It's too late to help Evan, but it's not too late to protect other young adults. It tears my heart apart when I hear about students dying from meningitis or suffering long-term disabilities. I want these young people to live full lives and fulfill their dreams.

"Give parents and students the information. I know they will make the choice to be immunized. Universities, healthcare providers, parents, and students all need to be educated about the vaccine.

"To me, there is nothing more precious than my children. I would do anything I could to protect them. That choice was not given to me. Give that choice to others. It would be a fitting tribute to Evan that, on this 18-month anniversary of his death, a recommendation for the vaccine be approved."

---

## THE MENINGOCOCCAL VACCINE

### What is the meningococcal vaccine, and how effective is it?

Like the pneumococcal vaccine for seniors, meningococcal vaccine is not live; it is a complex sugar from the microbe's cell wall. Four types of meningococcus are in the vaccine (A, C, Y, and W-135), but unfortunately these four represent only about half of the reported meningococcal infections in the U.S. As previously mentioned, the vaccine is not effective in children less than 2 years old.

Generally, only one dose of meningococcal vaccine is needed because the duration of risk is limited, but persons at continued high risk for infection may benefit from a second dose three to five years after the first. The effectiveness of the vaccine is short-lived, plummeting during the first three years after vaccination and even more rapidly in infants and young children.

### Who should get the vaccine?

**College students.** As mentioned above, because disease rates are slightly higher among college dormitory residents than among the general public, the

ACIP recommends that immunizations should be made available especially to freshmen. The American College Health Association had established this policy in 1997, urging college health services to take "a more proactive role in alerting students and their parents about the dangers of meningococcal disease" and in making sure that "all students have access to a vaccination program."

**Others.** While use of the vaccine is usually restricted to persons who are at least 2 years old, some short-term protection against type A can be obtained for infants as young as 3 months.

ACIP recommends use of the vaccine by three groups:

✛ Persons with medical conditions that make it difficult to fight off meningococcus (HIV infection, absent or nonfunctional spleen, terminal complement component deficiency).

✛ Research, industrial, and clinical laboratory personnel who routinely are exposed to meningococcus in solutions that may be aerosolized.

✛ Travelers and U.S. citizens residing in countries where the germ is common or where there is an epidemic. This is especially important if the traveler will have prolonged contact with local persons. The area with the highest rates is sub-Saharan Africa from the west coast to Ethiopia, especially during the dry season from December to June. Epidemics have occurred recently in Saudi Arabia, Kenya, Tanzania, Burundi, and Mongolia. Revaccination should be considered for those who have a persistent or recurring risk of meningococcal disease.

## Who should *not* get the vaccine?

Meningococcal disease vaccine should not be given to anyone who

✛ Is less than 2 years of age.

✛ Had a serious allergic reaction to a prior dose of meningococcal vaccine.

✛ Has a moderate to severe illness. If this is the case, the person may receive the vaccine when feeling better.

## What are the vaccine risks and side effects?

Allergic reactions could occur after any vaccine. Pain at the injection site is the most commonly reported adverse reaction. Pain or tenderness, swelling, or warmth at the injection site may occur in more than 40 percent of persons who receive the vaccine and may last one to two days. About 1 or 2 out of 100 young children will have fever.

## WHAT OTHER QUESTIONS DO PARENTS ASK?

*Q: My child is a leaving for college this fall. Should she get the meningococcal vaccine?*

College freshmen living in dormitories have five times higher rates of this disease than those who live in the community, but even in this group the risk is not much greater than 5 per 100,000. Neither the ACIP nor the American College Health Association specifically recommends meningococcal vaccine for this group; they just suggest that students and families be made aware of its availability. Because the vaccine is safe, fairly effective, and not outrageously expensive, many families are choosing to get it for their college-bound young adults.

## WHAT DOES THE FUTURE HOLD?

Scientists are working on a meningitis vaccine that will be more effective in infants. A new conjugate vaccine for type C meningococcus, which will work for infants, is already being used in the United Kingdom. Such a vaccine is not licensed in the U.S., but it is expected by 2002 to 2004.

Type B meningococcus causes a significant proportion of the invasive meningococcal disease in the U.S., but it is not represented in the current vaccine. Scientists have developed a vaccine that is safe and effective against type B in older children and adults, but this vaccine is not effective in children younger than 4 years old. No time estimates are available for the licensure of this vaccine.

*You'll always stay young if you live honestly, eat slowly, sleep sufficiently, work industriously, worship faithfully—and lie about your age.*

—Anonymous

# Chapter 18

# Vaccines for Adolescents and Adults:
## Td, Chickenpox, MMR, and Hepatitis B

**According to Dr. David Satcher,** the U.S. Surgeon General, in the late 1990s an estimated 45,000 adults died each year in the U.S. from influenza, pneumococcus, and hepatitis B—all of which are vaccine-preventable diseases. About 90 percent of all flu-associated deaths in the United States occur in persons aged 65 and older, and pneumococcal disease in this age group has an 80 percent death rate.

If adults stayed current on their immunizations, then death rates would drop. Although immunization rates in the U.S. are at an all-time high for people 65 and older (66 percent for influenza and 45 percent for pneumococcal vaccine as of 1997), these immunization rates are far lower than for children. Immunization of adults and adolescents with high-risk medical conditions lags even further behind.

In each disease chapter, when applicable, we have addressed the vaccine recommendations for adolescents and adults. In this chapter we focus solely on these age groups to remind teenagers, adults, parents, and grandparents that they need to be aware of new vaccines or boosters.

Note that routinely recommended vaccines are covered by the Vaccines for Children Program and so are free for many persons before their nineteenth birthday. Flu and pneumococcal vaccines are covered by Medicare, as is hepatitis B vaccine for some people.

## ALL ADOLESCENTS AND ADULTS

Persons aged 11 through 111 should be aware of the following vaccines.

**Hepatitis B vaccine.** If you are 11 to 18 years old, you should be sure to have received all three doses of the hepatitis B vaccine. Of course, if you are older than 18 and at increased risk for hepatitis B, you also should receive the vaccine. (See Chapter 8.)

**Tetanus and diphtheria (Td) vaccine.** If you never before had tetanus and diphtheria vaccines, you will need one dose now, a second dose one month later, and a third dose six months after the second dose. Subsequently, all adults need a booster dose every ten years.

The first Td booster can be given at 11 to 12 years of age and then every 10 years after that. It may help you remember the Td boosters if you get them around birthdays when you change decades, such as when you turn 20, 30, or 40 years old and so on. (See Chapter 9.)

**Measles, mumps, and rubella (MMR) vaccine.** If you were born after 1956, you should make sure that you are current for MMR. Like chickenpox, measles and mumps are particularly dangerous if contracted in adulthood. Having received the full series of MMR is especially important for college students, women who plan to become pregnant, persons working at a healthcare facility, persons traveling abroad, and persons born in countries where MMR was not given during childhood (unless they already had the diseases). Women who are planning to become pregnant should see below. (See Chapter 12.)

**Chickenpox vaccine.** Chickenpox can be a dangerous disease, especially for those who catch it later in life. If you already had the disease, even a mild case of it, you do not need the vaccine. If you are not sure that you had the disease, it is worth either getting the vaccine or having a blood test to see if you are immune and following up with vaccination if you are not. This is especially important for persons who live or work in settings where the virus can be spread (such as schools, daycare, institutional settings, or travel abroad). Women who are planning to become pregnant should see below. (See Chapter 13.)

**Meningococcus vaccine.** Due to the slightly higher risk of contracting meningococcus, freshmen dormitory residents should consider receiving a single dose of this vaccine. Check with your family physician or your college's student health services for information on this vaccine. (See Chapter 17.)

## WOMEN OF CHILDBEARING AGE

Women of childbearing age should be sure they are immune to **rubella** (German measles) and **chickenpox.** It is very important for women to get these vaccines if they are not already immune. Because of the theoretical possibility of damage to a fetus, ACIP recommends that women avoid becoming pregnant for one month after receiving the chickenpox vaccine and for three months after receiving the rubella vaccine.

If you are pregnant, you also should be aware of the following vaccines.

**Flu vaccine.** If you will be in the second or third trimester of pregnancy during flu season, which usually peaks from December to March in the U.S., you should receive the flu vaccine in the fall. If you are pregnant and have a high-risk medical condition, you should be vaccinated before flu season regardless of your stage of pregnancy. (See Chapter 16.)

**Hepatitis B vaccine.** If you are not already immune to hepatitis B and are at risk for hepatitis B (see Chapter 8 for details), you should receive the vaccine as soon as possible.

**Tetanus and diphtheria (Td) vaccine.** If you have not had the Td booster in more than nine years, you should receive one any time during pregnancy. Having active antibodies against tetanus and diphtheria will protect your newborn because you will pass the antibodies to the fetus. (See Chapter 9.)

## HEALTHCARE WORKERS

Doctors, nurses, nursing aides, and anyone else in the healthcare field should be current on the following vaccines.

**Hepatitis B vaccine.** Two hundred healthcare workers die each year in the U.S. from hepatitis B. You should receive this vaccine series if you have any chance of being exposed to blood or blood-contaminated body fluids. (Ask yourself if you're willing to bet your life that every single person you work with has properly disposed of every needle, carefully cleaned every blood spatter, etc.) One to two months after having received the series of three hepatitis B vaccinations, take a blood test to make sure you have become immune. If you have not become immune after three doses, you should receive further hepatitis B vaccination. (See Chapter 8.)

**MMR vaccine.** If you were born before 1957 or if you've had blood tests that show you are immune to all three viruses, you don't need the vaccine. Otherwise, you should be sure you've had two doses. (See Chapter 12.)

**Chickenpox vaccine.** Chickenpox is especially bad if you catch it as an adult. As a healthcare worker, you really don't want to spread it to patients—especially if they are infants, elderly, or immuno-compromised. If you already had the disease, even a mild case, you do not need the vaccine. If you are not sure, either get the vaccine or have a blood test to see if you are immune, and then follow up with vaccination if you are not. (See Chapter 13.)

**Flu vaccine.** You should receive this vaccine if you come in contact with someone who could become seriously ill if he or she were exposed to flu virus. This includes everyone 50 and older, residents of a nursing home, and persons with long-term illnesses. (See Chapter 16 and below).

## Older Adults and Those in Nursing Homes

**Flu vaccine.** If you are 50 or older, you should receive this every year between September and mid-November, without fail.

**Pneumococcal vaccine.** If you are 65 or older, you should receive this vaccine. People with a chronic illness or a weakened immune system need two doses five years apart. Everyone else can receive a single dose.

## Persons with Long-term Illness or a Weakened Immune System

Persons who have a long-term illness (such as heart, lung, blood, or kidney disease; diabetes; or cancer) or a weakened immune system (from treatment with X rays or medications, HIV, a damaged spleen, and so on) should talk to their physician about the following vaccines.

**Hib vaccine.** In addition to flu and pneumococcal vaccines, if you have an absent or poorly functioning spleen or a weakened immune system, you should receive Hib vaccine.

**MMR and chickenpox vaccines.** If you have HIV, you should receive MMR and chickenpox vaccines if (a) you are not already immune to these diseases and (b) you are not severely immunosuppressed (that is, you are HIV positive, but you have no symptoms of AIDS).

**Pneumococcal vaccine.** If you have a long-term illness, you should receive two doses of this vaccine separated by five years. Persons with liver disease, alcoholism, or spinal fluid leaks should also receive pneumococcal vaccine. Asthma is not an indication for pneumococcal vaccine.

**Flu vaccine.** You should receive the flu vaccine every year between September and mid-November, without fail. Also, if you have asthma, you should receive flu vaccine.

## PERSONS AT RISK FOR HEPATITIS B AND HEPATITIS A

**Hepatitis B vaccine.** Persons at increased risk for hepatitis B should receive the vaccine. The risk groups include, for example, healthcare workers who handle blood or needles, persons who receive blood products (hemodialysis, hemophilia), heterosexuals who have more than one partner, homosexual males, and injection drug users. (See Chapter 8 for details.)

**Hepatitis A vaccine.** Persons at increased risk for hepatitis A should receive the vaccine. Because hepatitis A is spread through human stools and rarely through blood, the risk groups relate to age (young children and persons caring for them), regions of the U.S. (persons living in some of the western and plains states), race/ethnicity and poverty (persons who are poor, who live in unsanitary conditions, or who are from Central or South America or other developing countries), and increased exposure to blood or stool (patients receiving blood clotting factors, homosexual males, and illicit drug users). (See Chapter 14 for details.)

## OTHER VACCINES

Other vaccines are recommended for adolescents and adults who risk exposure to certain diseases. Please refer to the chapters on Meningococcus (17), Special Circumstances (19), Travelers (20), Bioterrorism (21), and Future Vaccines (22).

*In its beginning the malady [tuberculosis] is easier to cure but difficult to detect; but later it becomes easy to detect but difficult to cure.*

—Niccolo Machiavelli

# Chapter 19

# Vaccines for Special Circumstances:
## Lyme Disease, Rabies, and Tuberculosis

Relatively few Americans need the vaccines against Lyme disease, rabies, or tuberculosis (TB). However, when indicated, these vaccines may prevent significant disease and suffering. Parents wonder if their children should receive the Lyme disease vaccine, which is quite new and has received some attention in the media. Questions about rabies vaccine enter the minds of every parent whose child is bitten by an animal, and should enter the minds of some international travelers. Tuberculosis is confusing for many U.S. parents because they mistakenly believe their children received a TB vaccine, when in reality the injection they received was a test for TB. Each of these diseases and the vaccines that prevent them are explained below.

## LYME DISEASE

Two mothers contacted their state health department in 1975 about the high number of children in their Lyme, Connecticut, neighborhood who were developing joint inflammation. Many had been diagnosed with juvenile rheumatoid arthritis, but this uncommon disease was not known to occur in clusters. The report led to an investigation and, ultimately, to the first identification of Lyme disease. Between 1993 and 1997, approximately 12,500 cases of Lyme disease were reported annually in the United States.

## What is Lyme disease, and how is it spread?

A corkscrew-shaped microbe, *Borrelia burgdorferi,* causes Lyme disease. Deer ticks—small ticks that usually feed on deer, mice, and birds—carry the bacterium and spread it to humans they bite. In the U.S., most cases of Lyme disease are restricted to the northeast, the mid-Atlantic, the upper north-central states, and northwestern California. (See Figure 19-1.)

Ticks tend to live near the ground in moist, shaded areas, particularly in tall grasses, leaf litter, overgrown brush, and woody environments. So people who frequent these areas are at risk, especially from June to August when young ticks are feeding. Children less than 10 years of age and middle-aged adults (possibly because so many work outside or garden) are most likely to contract Lyme disease.

**Figure 19-1**
## AREAS AT RISK FOR LYME DISEASE

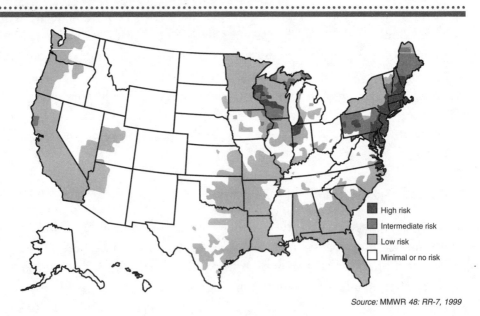

*Source:* MMWR *48: RR-7, 1999*

The most consistent finding is the initial skin lesion. It is a red patch or pimple that expands around a tick bite—though only a few patients recall experiencing a tick bite. Often, the center of the patch returns almost to its normal color, so the patch looks like a bull's eye (pale in the middle, ringed in red). The sore may become quite large, exceeding five centimeters across. Sixty to 80 percent of persons with Lyme disease develop this skin lesion.

Patients may develop a host of flu-like symptoms, including swollen or painful joints and muscle aches. Some patients go on to develop a strange rash three to five weeks later, along with inflammation of the brain or its outer cover (meningitis), paralysis of the facial muscles, or conduction defects in the heart.

### What is the treatment for Lyme disease?

Many oral antibiotics are available to treat Lyme disease. Specific regimens are prescribed depending on the symptoms, and 75 to 80 percent of persons treated will recover from the disease. Unfortunately, before treatment some patients will develop a severe case of the disease, with tissue damage and disability.

To avoid being bitten by the deer tick you should use outdoor insecticides and keep deer away from areas where children play (use an eight-foot-high or electrified fence). However, personal protection measures are often more realistic. These include the following:

✚ Wear light-colored clothing to make ticks more visible.

✚ Tuck pant legs into socks to keep ticks off your legs.

✚ Use tick or insect repellents (e.g., DEET on skin or clothes, permethrin on clothes only).

✚ Conduct daily inspections of children and pets for attached ticks. (Ticks on a person for less than 48 hours probably won't transmit the disease.)

✚ If a tick bite sore begins to widen, seek medical advice.

### What is the Lyme disease vaccine, and how effective is it?

The Lyme disease vaccine is inactivated, being a protein piece of the microbe's cell wall. The vaccine was licensed in the U.S. in 1998 for persons age 15 to 70 years of age. Testing in children younger than 15 is not yet complete, so to prevent tick bites, parents should make sure their children follow the precautions listed above.

Three doses of Lyme disease vaccine are needed. The first two doses are given one month apart; the third dose follows the first by 12 months. The second and third doses should be timed to be given before April, the beginning of the tick season. After three doses, the vaccine is effective for more than 75 percent of the people who received it.

### Who should get the vaccine?

ACIP recommends that you consider getting the vaccine if you are 15 to 70 years old and

+ Live, work, or play in an area of high or medium risk for Lyme disease (see map); *and*

+ Are in tick-infested areas often or for long periods.

You may consider getting the vaccine if you spend less time in tick areas.

### Who should *not* get the vaccine?

Lyme disease vaccine should not be given to anyone who
+ Is less than 15 or more than 70 years old.

+ Had a serious allergic reaction to a prior dose of Lyme disease vaccine.

+ Has a moderate to severe illness. If this is the case, the person may receive the vaccine when feeling better.

## What are the vaccine risks and side effects?

Allergic reactions could occur after any vaccine. Pain or tenderness, swelling, or warmth at the injection site may occur in about 25 percent of people who receive the vaccine and last one to two days. About 3 percent of people will have muscle or joint aches, flu-like symptoms, fever, or chills.

## What other questions do people ask?

*Q: We are going on vacation to an area that is known for Lyme disease and we are camping out. Everyone in our family has gotten the vaccine except the person who rolls around in the bushes the most: my 8-year-old son. Why shouldn't he get the vaccine?*

Tests of vaccine safety and effectiveness are not complete for children younger than 15, so preventing tick bites is the recommended alternative until a vaccine becomes available.

## RABIES

The World Health Organization estimates that, worldwide, 3 million people are vaccinated each year after exposure to rabies. Back in 1983, rabies killed 50,000 persons. Now more than 50 countries are free of rabies, but travelers staying more than 30 days in rabies-infested countries should get the vaccine (or avoid stray animals).

In the United States between 1980 and 1996, only 32 people were diagnosed with rabies, averaging one to two per year, although four deaths were reported in the U.S. in 1997. Each year in the U.S., an estimated 18,000 persons receive pre-exposure vaccine and 40,000 receive post-exposure treatment. Even though the number of persons exposed to rabies each year is relatively small, the horror of the symptoms and the inevitability of death without vaccination or treatment make rabies a dreaded disease.

## What is rabies disease, and how is it spread?

Rabies virus is common among wild animals, but usually is only a threat to humans when an infected animal bites a human. The virus enters the body, attaches to the distant nerve endings, and follows the connection of nerves to the brain. It may take as little as six days or as long as six years for the virus to reach the brain, but usually the incubation phase is a month or two.

A preliminary illness follows in which the patient has a headache, fever, fatigue, and a loss of appetite. The rabies-infected person may have intermittent spurts of irritability, aggression, viciousness, and hyper-reactivity to light, touch, or sound. Attempts to eat or drink—and, eventually, the mere sight of liquids—may produce painful throat spasms, causing the patient to develop a fear of water (hydrophobia). Increased saliva output and the inability to swallow give the patient the appearance of "foaming at the mouth."

More central nervous symptoms, such as convulsions, may appear before the next phase, in which the muscles of the head and neck—including those responsible for speaking and breathing—and of one or more limbs become weak or paralyzed. Death from rabies may be sudden or preceded by coma for hours or months.

Humans usually catch the rabies virus from animal bites or other exposure to infected saliva, but it can also be contracted through inhalation of contaminated air (such as that in caves with a lot of bat droppings). Wild animals—raccoons, skunks, bats, and foxes—are the most frequent carriers of rabies, and contact with them accounts for 92 percent of the reported cases in Americans in recent years. Domestic animals—dogs, cats, and cattle—account for 7 percent of rabies cases in humans in the U.S. Worldwide, rabid dogs account for more than 90 percent of cases of humans exposed to rabies.

Human rabies is most common in children younger than age 15, with the highest incidence in rural boys during summer months.

### What is the treatment for rabies?

Medical care should be sought immediately. Thorough and careful wound cleansing is essential. If the bitten person has not previously been vaccinated against rabies, then he or she should receive the series of six injections. Once symptoms develop, no vaccine or medication improves the person's chance of survival. (Only seven humans are known to have survived rabies once symptoms set in.)

## What is the rabies vaccine, and how effective is it?

Rabies vaccine contains killed rabies virus. The vaccine is recommended as a three-dose series over 28 days if used *before* an exposure. Boosters are needed if the risk persists. *After* an exposure, rabies vaccine should be given immediately with immune globulin and then five subsequent doses are spaced over 28 days. When given according to the ACIP recommendations, the regime is almost 100 percent effective.

## Who should get the vaccine?

**Before a rabies exposure.** If you will be in settings where you will be exposed to animals and where you might not have immediate access to good healthcare, you should consider getting the rabies vaccine before an exposure. (Even if you get rabies vaccine before an exposure, you would still need two doses of vaccine if you were bitten by a rabid animal.)

ACIP does not strongly recommend the rabies vaccine for U.S. residents. *Pre-exposure* vaccination should be *offered* to persons in high-risk groups, such as veterinarians, animal handlers, and certain lab workers, and it should be *considered* for others with frequent contact with potentially rabid bats, raccoons, skunks, cats, dogs, or other potentially rabid animals. ACIP states that international travelers might be candidates if they are likely to come in contact with animals in areas where dog rabies is common and the likelihood of immediate healthcare (including rabies vaccine and immune globulin) is limited.

**After a rabies exposure.** The decision to start treatment *after* a possible exposure is complicated and important. In addition to the type of exposure, the animal's species, general health, and availability for 10 days of observation must be factored in. Your physician may need to consult local or state public health officials for guidance.

## Who should *not* get the vaccine?

✚ Persons with a serious allergic response to rabies vaccine should be revaccinated with caution.

✛ Persons who have an immune system weakened by medicines
(such as chemotherapy, prednisone) or illness (such as cancer,
HIV) should be aware that the vaccine may be ineffective for
them. They should avoid activities that put them at risk until
their immune system is better able to respond to the vaccine. If
high-risk activities cannot be avoided, the vaccine may be given
before exposure, but antibody levels should be checked to see if
the vaccine worked.

## What are the vaccine risks and side effects?

The current rabies vaccines have fewer side effects than the old vaccines.
About 25 percent of persons who receive the vaccine will have some itching, swelling, redness, or pain at the injection site. Another 20 percent will
have headache, muscle aches, nausea, or dizziness. Between day 2 and 21,
about 6 percent of persons who receive the booster dose will develop hives,
sometimes with nausea, vomiting, fever, or joint symptoms.

## What other questions do people ask?

*Q: I have always heard that rabies shots had to be given in the stomach. Is
this true?*

This is not true. Rabies vaccine should be given in the upper arm muscle
of older children and adults, and the outer thigh muscle of younger children.

# TUBERCULOSIS (TB)

Tuberculosis, or TB, is probably responsible for more human death in
Europe and the United States than any other infection in recorded history.
Worldwide, TB infects one out of three persons. Each year 8 million people
become ill with TB, and 2 to 3 million die of it. Compared with technologically advanced areas, developing countries bear a greater and increasing TB
burden.

In 1998 in the United States, 18,000 cases of active TB were reported,
down 8 percent from 1997. This was the sixth year in a row that the num-

ber of active TB cases declined since the 1980s, when the number of cases had begun to increase. The high prevalence of tuberculosis in developing countries, combined with frequent travel to and from all countries, has increased the proportion of cases among persons in the U.S. who were foreign born, from 27 percent of all reported U.S. cases in 1992 to 42 percent in 1998.

## What is tuberculosis, and how is it spread?

*Mycobacterium tuberculosis* is a member of a large family of bacteria. It is transmitted from one person to another when a multitude of tiny mucus droplets fly from the nose or mouth of an infected person who coughs, sneezes, or speaks. When the bacteria invade the human body, most persons' immune systems can contain it, so the disease remains latent. However, the immune systems of 5 to 10 percent of those infected with the disease cannot fight it, and the disease becomes active.

Active TB usually manifests as lung disease that can range from mild cough with a shortness of breath to severe cough with high spiking fevers and night sweats. The body tries to wall off the infection, but these walled off areas can rupture, spilling infected pus around the lungs or heart. If the bacteria invade the central nervous system or spread throughout the body, death usually follows.

In the U.S., the chief strategy against TB is twofold: Prevent TB transmission from persons who have active TB and prevent latent TB from turning into active TB. Both of these require early detection and treatment. Early detection and treatment are especially important in settings where TB infection is common or carries the most risk, for example, in settings where HIV-infected people receive healthcare.

Each year in the United States in the mid-1800s, about 400 out of 100,000 people in eastern states died from TB. By 1900 that number was down to 200 out of 100,000 and by 1950 it was 26 out of 100,000. This improvement was not due to antibiotics or vaccines, but to better social conditions. Now, TB is not common in the general U.S. population, and almost 60 percent of all cases in 1994, for example, were reported in just five states (California, Florida, Illinois, New York, and Texas).

Among people who have normal immune systems, those at greatest risk of developing active TB are poor, undernourished, have poor access to healthcare, and live in crowded conditions. In Western nations three groups are at increased risk: elderly whites, young adults and children from racial or ethnic minorities, and foreign-born immigrants.

The greatest risk factor for progressing from latent to active TB is a weakened immune system, especially if weakened by HIV. While 5 to 10 percent of otherwise healthy adults infected with TB will develop the active disease *in their lifetimes,* 5 to 10 percent of persons infected with both HIV and TB will develop active TB disease *each year.*

### What is the treatment for TB?

Antibiotics are available to treat and prevent TB. Three or four medicines must be taken faithfully for several months. As anyone who has tried to stick to an antibiotic regime even for a short time can appreciate, taking a number of antibiotics for long periods is not easy. Often special arrangements must be made to make sure that a patient keeps to the schedule. Unfortunately, a growing number of TB infections are resistant to one or more antibiotics. Resistant strains must be treated with more medications and the regime is longer.

### What is the TB vaccine, and how effective is it?

TB vaccine, known as BCG, is a live but weakened cousin of *M. tuberculosis.* It was first administered to humans in 1921. New TB vaccines are being developed in the hope that a more effective vaccine will be found.

Indeed, BCG is not used routinely in the U.S. in part because the vaccine is not particularly effective at preventing infection. A summary of relatively recent studies showed BCG was about 75 to 86 percent effective in preventing life-threatening forms of TB in children. Another summary of studies showed BCG was about 50 percent effective against all TB. Many questions remain unanswered about the usefulness of the vaccine for adolescents and adults, healthcare workers, and patients with HIV infection.

## Who should get the vaccine?

The vaccine is rarely recommended in the United States because its effectiveness is questionable. Also, the vaccine makes the skin test for TB hard to interpret, which in turn makes it difficult to reliably identify persons who are infected with TB.

Almost all children who catch TB get it from an adult. If an infant or child is (1) continually exposed to a patient with infectious TB of the lungs *and* (2) not already infected with TB, the vaccine should be considered under certain circumstances. These include

- The TB patient is untreated or ineffectively treated and the child can neither be separated from the patient nor given long-term preventive medicines.

- The TB patient has a strain that is resistant to antibiotics and the child cannot be separated from the patient.

The vaccine should also be considered for some healthcare workers.

## Who should *not* get the vaccine?

The following persons should not receive the vaccine:

- Those who have had a severe allergic or systemic reaction following a prior dose of TB vaccine or any of its components.

- Those who have a moderate or severe acute illness should postpone vaccination until they have recovered from that illness.

- Those who have a weakened immune system for any reason, including HIV.

- Those who have a positive reaction to a TB skin test.

- Pregnant women. No harmful effects to the fetus have been associated with BCG vaccine, but its use is not recommended during pregnancy.

### What are the vaccine risks and side effects?

Allergic reactions could occur after any vaccine. Pain, redness, or swelling are common after BCG. Two reactions that are not uncommon after BCG and that may last for as long as three months include the following:

✚ Moderate swelling of the lymph nodes in the armpits or neck. In some people, this may progress to pus-filled nodes that require drainage.

✚ Swelling at the site of the injection, which may turn into a pustule and then a scar. In some people, an ulcer may develop where the shot was given.

The BCG vaccine for TB is a live germ, and although it is weakened, some people cannot fight it off. They may die from infection throughout the body. Fatal disseminated disease has been reported in 1.9 to 15.6 per 10 million vaccinated infants and in 0.6 to 7.2 per 10 million vaccinated persons ages 1 to 20.

### What other questions do people ask?

*Q: My family is traveling to Africa. Should my child (and I) receive the TB vaccine before we leave?*
The BCG vaccine is not indicated for a U.S. resident traveling abroad.

*Q. Should testing for TB be part of my child's routine well-child care?*
Yes. TB skin testing is performed at the 9-month well-child visit if the family has any of the following risk factors: low socio-economic status, residence in an area where TB is present, exposure to TB, or immigration from a high-risk country. The TB skin test is performed at the 12- or 15-month well-child visit before or with the MMR vaccine.

*For my part, I travel not to go anywhere, but to go. I travel for travel's sake. The great affair is to move.*

—Robert Louis Stevenson

# Chapter 20

# Vaccines for Traveling Abroad:
## Cholera, Japanese Encephalitis, Plague, Typhoid, and Yellow Fever

The vaccinations that you and your family might need depend on which countries you will be traveling to, what parts of those countries you plan to visit (such as tourist sites or remote areas), how long you plan to stay in those areas, and how old the members of your family are. If you are planning a trip, we offer these tips.

First, start planning early, at least eight weeks before departing. As soon as you know your destination, ask your healthcare provider or local health department which vaccines (and other preventive measures) you might need. Some vaccine series take months to complete, and many travelers make the mistake of waiting until the last minute.

Second, don't neglect routine immunization before going abroad. Before leaving the U.S., your child (and you) should be up-to-date on MMR, polio, and chickenpox vaccines. You should also consider hepatitis A, flu, meningococcus, and rabies. The risk of catching these infectious diseases is much higher in some areas, not to mention in airplanes and on cruise liners where large numbers of people are in close quarters and possibly coming from a place where disease is prevalent.

Third, keep detailed records of all vaccines that your family has received, including travel vaccines, so you are prepared for your next trip.

If your healthcare provider's office does not have detailed information, your state or local health department is usually a good place to turn to next. Often these departments have a travel health specialist on staff. Also, you can contact the following agencies:

- ✚ Centers for Disease Control and Prevention, via fax at 888-232-3299, or online at http://www.cdc.gov/travel

- ✚ International Society of Travel Medicine, http://www.istm.org (includes a directory of U.S. travel clinics)

- ✚ American Society of Tropical Medicine and Hygiene, http://www.astmh.org (also includes a directory of U.S. travel clinics)

- ✚ Pan American Health Organization (PAHO, a Western Hemisphere office of the World Health Organization), http://www.paho.org (includes country-specific health information)

- ✚ World Health Organization, http://www.who.org (provides disease surveillance data worldwide)

- ✚ International Association for Medical Assistance to Travelers at 716-754-4883. This organization has a directory of English-speaking doctors.

- ✚ American Citizens Services at 202-647-5225. They offer medical, financial, and legal assistance for American travelers abroad.

## CHOLERA

### What is cholera, how is it spread, and how is it treated?

Cholera is caused by bacteria, *Vibrio cholerae*, that contaminate water or food, especially fish or shellfish. Persons can avoid cholera by not eating raw or undercooked food and by not drinking water that has not been boiled, filtered, or chemically disinfected. (Ice cubes in drinks often are made from untreated water.) Cholera is common in Central and South America, Asia, and Africa. Usually the disease occurs in areas of poverty, not in tourist sites where facilities and funds are available to treat the water and to prepare the food more carefully. About 1 in 500,000 returning Western travelers report getting cholera.

One to three days after exposure, the poison produced by the cholera bacteria will give infected persons diarrhea, often with vomiting but without fever. Only 2 to 5 percent of infections are severe, but cholera can lead to a rapid and life-threatening loss of fluids and body salts. Because the bacteria are killed by stomach acids, few persons get sick with cholera unless they ingest a large amount of the bacteria in a heavily contaminated source or their stomach acids have been diminished by antacids or anti-ulcer medications. Others at risk include persons with liver disease or immunodeficiency.

The main treatment is large amounts of rehydrating fluids. Oral rehydration solution (ORS), prepared from packets of rehydration salts distributed by the World Health Organization, is the best fluid to drink because it contains the optimal mix of body salts. (ORS packets are available in the U.S. from Jianas Brothers Packaging Company, Kansas City, MO; telephone 816-421-2880.) Commercial rehydration products, such as Pedialyte™, are also effective but are bulky to pack. Of course, if the patient vomits all the fluids taken by mouth, then intravenous fluids may be needed.

Persons who have moderate to severe cholera can take antibiotics to shorten the course of the illness. The cholera bacteria, however, are becoming increasingly resistant to some of the common antibiotics.

## How effective is the cholera vaccine, and who should get it?

The cholera vaccine protects only about 50 percent of the persons who are injected with it, and it is completely ineffective against some strains of the bacteria. Two doses are recommended for people at highest risk and should be given one week to one month or more apart. Boosters are necessary every six months if the risk of disease persists. Protection starts about two weeks after the second dose.

Luckily, the risk of cholera is so low that the vaccine is not recommended for U.S. travelers. And no country currently requires cholera vaccine for entry. Despite World Health Organization recommendations, however, local authorities in some areas (such as in Africa) demand proof of cholera vaccination or a medical exemption certificate for entry. If you have neither of these, you may be faced with having your itinerary rearranged abruptly or with border patrol offering on-the-spot single dose cholera vaccination (which greatly increases your risk of HIV and hepatitis B). Some travel experts suggest that vaccination or official exemption may be advisable if you are going to or through an African country where cholera is active.

The cholera vaccine may be of benefit for three groups of international travelers:

✛ Persons taking antacids or anti-ulcer medications (such as Zantac™, Tagamet™, Prevacid™, Prilosec™). Remember that stomach acids are the best line of defense when contaminated food or drink is consumed.

✛ Persons who will be in areas of poor sanitation for a prolonged time (such as famine relief workers in refugee camps in endemic areas).

✛ Persons traveling to areas where there is no prompt access to reliable medical care (such as backpackers).

## Who should *not* get the vaccine?

Persons with a history of a severe allergic or systemic reaction following a prior dose of cholera vaccine or any of its components should not take cholera vaccine.

Others who should avoid the vaccine include the following:

✛ Persons who have a moderate or severe acute illness. These individuals should postpone vaccination.

✛ Children less than 6 months old. (For older children the dose and route of cholera vaccine is age-dependent. Seek advice from a knowledgeable healthcare provider.)

✛ Pregnant women. A pregnant woman should only receive the cholera vaccine if it is clearly needed.

## What are the vaccine risks and side effects?

Cholera vaccination is associated with more local side effects than most other vaccines. Most persons experience pain, swelling, and redness at the cholera vaccine injection site. This may begin soon after the shot and usually resolves within a few days. Frequently persons experience malaise, headache, and mild to moderate fever for a day or two after cholera vaccine. Severe allergic reactions and other severe reactions occur rarely after cholera vaccine.

## Additional notes

✛ Vaccination for yellow fever and cholera should be separated by at least three weeks because these vaccines interfere with each other.

✛ Plague vaccine and the injectable typhoid vaccine often cause side effects similar to the cholera vaccine. Theoretically, getting these vaccines at the same time could lead to a bigger reaction. If you have time, you may be more comfortable if you separate vaccinations by a week or more before leaving.

✛ Cholera vaccines that are taken by mouth are more effective. Though available in several other countries, they are not licensed in the U.S.

✛ Mutachol is a drug available in Canada, Europe, and Latin America that is 86 percent effective in preventing any diarrhea from cholera, and it is well tolerated. It is produced by Berna Pharmaceuticals.

## JAPANESE ENCEPHALITIS

### What is Japanese encephalitis, how is it spread, and how is it treated?

Japanese encephalitis (JE) is inflammation of the brain caused by a virus that is spread by a bite from the culex mosquito.

Within 5 to 15 days of the mosquito bite, symptoms will develop that range from headache and fever to lethargy and may include vomiting, diarrhea, seizure, or coma. Only 1 out of 250 infected persons have any symptoms, but 5 to 30 percent of persons who develop symptoms die. Also, 30 to 50 percent of survivors have some permanent damage to their central nervous system such as paralysis, convulsions, memory loss, or behavioral disturbances. The only treatment for JE is supportive care.

From 1978 to 1992, only 11 cases of JE were reported in U.S. citizens living or traveling in Asia, and at least 6 of these cases were soldiers living in field conditions. Fewer than 1 in 1 million unvaccinated American tourists in Asia have contracted JE. Those persons who lived in conditions of intense exposure for a month during peak transmission season increased their risk to 1 in 5,000.

Many factors determine the risk of contracting JE, including the region of the world, the habitat, the season, and even the time of day. JE is reported in Southeast Asia, India, China, Japan, and Korea (see Figure 20-1). The mosquitoes that spread JE often live where they have plenty of water to breed in and domestic animals, especially pigs, to feed upon. The mosquitoes feed in the evening and at night. So, to some extent, Japanese encephalitis can be prevented by avoiding rural-agricultural, rice-growing, pig-farming regions of Asia once the sun has gone down. The right conditions for spread of the virus also exist near or within many Asian cities, but risk to travelers in these areas is very low.

Although JE is a threat year-round in tropical regions of Asia and Oceania, in most temperate areas transmission is highest from April to September. In northern India and Nepal, transmission peaks from June to November.

### How effective is the Japanese encephalitis vaccine, and who should get it?

Although it is difficult to determine how effective the vaccine is at protecting Western travelers, field testing with children in Taiwan showed the

**Figure 20-1**
## REGIONS AT RISK FOR JAPANESE ENCEPHALITIS

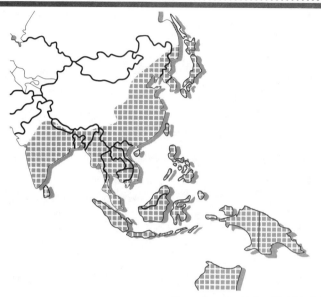

*Source: Based on data from World Health Organization, 1986–1998*

vaccine to be 80 percent effective. The ACIP recommends three doses: the second follows the first by 7 days and the third follows the first by 30 days. If departure is imminent, the third dose may follow the first by only 14 days. Just two doses given a week apart confer short-term immunity in 80 percent of vaccinees, but stopping there is not recommended. A booster is recommended two years after the initial series if the risk of disease persists. Protection starts about 10 days after the vaccine series.

The JE vaccine should be considered for travelers who will be in the risk areas of Asia, the Indian subcontinent, and the western Pacific for a month or longer. Persons who will be in these regions for a shorter period but intensively exposed to the mosquitoes may also benefit from vaccination.

## Who should *not* get the vaccine?

✛ Persons with a history of a severe allergic or systemic reaction following a prior dose of JE vaccine or any of its components should not receive this vaccine.

✛ Children less than 12 months old should not receive the vaccine.

✛ Persons with a moderate or severe acute illness should postpone vaccination.

✛ Pregnant women should avoid this vaccine. A pregnant woman should only receive the JE vaccine if the benefits outweigh the risks.

### What are the vaccine risks and side effects?

About 20 percent of vaccinated persons experience pain, swelling, and redness at the vaccine injection site. These symptoms may begin soon after the shot and usually resolve within a few days. About 10 percent of vaccinated persons experience malaise, fever, headache, rash, dizziness, muscle aches, vomiting, or abdominal pain.

Severe allergic reactions and other severe reactions occur rarely after JE vaccine. Such reactions usually begin within a day or two, but they may be delayed until a week to two after a second dose of vaccine. For this reason—and to ensure maximum protection—you should schedule the last dose of this vaccination series at least 10 days before departure.

### Additional notes

To minimize your risk when traveling to a JE-infected region during transmission season, wear mosquito repellent, wear a long-sleeved shirt and long pants, avoid outdoor activities in the evening, and sleep under permethrin-impregnated mosquito netting or in a screened or air-conditioned room.

## PLAGUE

### What is plague, how is it spread, and how is it treated?

In the mid-fourteenth century, a single infectious disease killed 25 to 30 percent of the European population and came to be known as the Black Death. Three such epidemics have been recorded, causing a death toll of 200 million (almost equal to the entire population of the United States today!).

This infectious disease, the plague, has not been eradicated. The most common form of plague is bubonic, meaning the lymph glands in the groin, armpit, and neck swell (that is, form buboes). The bubonic plague bacteria, *Yersinia pestis*, are carried by rats, other rodents, or less commonly, domestic animals such as cats. A person could catch the plague by handling an infected animal, but more commonly, the disease is spread when a flea that has bitten an infected animal later bites a human. It is also possible to catch the plague by inhaling droplets coughed by a person who has the plague. The symptoms of bubonic plague begin two to six days after exposure. Initial signs of plague are the same as those for a dozen other diseases: fever, chills, muscle aches, nausea, exhaustion, sore throat, and headache. Antibiotics taken early in the course of the disease are quite effective. If untreated, plague ends in death 50 to 60 percent of the time. The cause of death is the overwhelming inflammatory response that leads to breathing difficulties, clotting abnormalities, shock, and organ failure.

Wild rodents continue to carry plague in rural areas of the Americas (including the western third of the U.S.), Asia, and Africa, and southeastern Europe near the Caspian Sea, but plague rarely spreads to humans from

**Figure 20-2**
## DISTRIBUTION OF PLAGUE

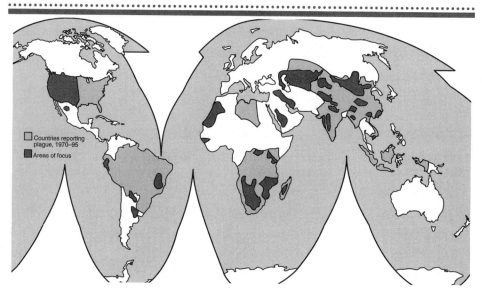

Countries reporting plague, 1970–95
Areas of focus

*Source: MMWR 45: RR-14, 1996*

them (see Figure 20-2). Urban outbreaks of plague—from rats living near humans—have been rare and relatively small over the past several decades. In fact, from 1980 to 1994, worldwide only just over 1,000 cases were reported each year on average. Usually, the disease occurs in areas of extreme poverty, not tourism.

Plague prevention really comes down to a few measures. In plague infected areas,

- ✛ Avoid the animals that carry plague (fleas, rats, rabbits, squirrels, chipmunks), especially if they are sick or dead.

- ✛ Make food and shelter inaccessible to rodents. Keep garbage covered.

- ✛ Regularly use flea powders on domestic animals.

- ✛ Use insect repellents on persons. Use insect repellent with DEET on exposed skin and repellent with permethrin on clothing.

- ✛ Use insecticides in home, recreational, and work environments when local animals or fleas have been found to be carrying plague.

- ✛ If you are at high risk of exposure, consider taking preventive antibiotics, such as doxycycline or tetracycline for adults and trimethoprim-sulfamethoxazole for children less than 10.

### How effective is plague vaccine, and who should get it?

Studies have not been done to directly measure the value of plague vaccine. The low incidence of plague among vaccinated U.S. military personnel exposed to plague in Vietnam suggests that the vaccine protects against flea-borne plague.

No country currently requires plague vaccine for entry. The ACIP recommends that only persons at very high risk should consider getting plague vaccine. Specifically, this includes lab workers who routinely deal with the bacteria and field workers who have regular contact with wild rodents or their fleas in plague-infected areas.

Two doses should be given one to three months apart. The third dose is given five to six months after dose two. For persons with ongoing exposure, boosters one, two, and three are given every six months; thereafter boosters should be given every year or two.

## Who should *not* get the vaccine?

✛ Persons with a history of a severe allergic or systemic reaction following a prior dose of plague vaccine or any of its components should not receive the vaccine.

✛ Persons with a moderate or severe acute illness should postpone vaccination.

✛ Children younger than 18 years old should not receive the vaccine.

✛ Pregnant women should avoid this vaccine. A pregnant woman should only receive the plague vaccine if it is clearly needed.

## What are the vaccine risks and side effects?

Plague vaccine produces more severe side effects than most vaccines, and repeated doses of the vaccine increase the probability of the side effects. About 30 percent of vaccine recipients experience pain, swelling, and redness at the plague vaccine injection site. This begins soon after the shot and usually resolves within two days. About 20 percent experience malaise, headache, fever, and swollen lymph glands for a day or two after receiving the plague vaccine. Severe allergic reactions and other moderate to severe reactions such as severe headache, joint pain, or shaking chills occur infrequently (about 4 in 1,000) after plague vaccine.

## Additional notes

Cholera vaccine and the injected typhoid vaccine often cause side effects much as plague vaccine does. Theoretically, getting these vaccines at the same time could lead to a bigger reaction. If you have time to separate these vaccinations by a week or more and still get all the vaccines you need before leaving, you may be more comfortable.

## Typhoid

### What is typhoid, how is it spread, and how is it treated?

Typhoid fever is caused by bacteria *(Salmonella typhi)* and usually manifests with a combination of fever, chills, headache, weakness, loss of appetite, abdominal pain, body aches, and cough. Small, red spots appear on the chest, abdomen, and back of about 20 percent of white patients. Constipation is common in older children and adults, but diarrhea may occur in younger children. The germ that causes typhoid fever can stay in the bloodstream or cause infections in the bones, liver, or lungs. Typhoid fever can cause a life-threatening perforation of the intestines and massive bleeding. Antibiotics are available to treat typhoid fever. Unfortunately, the disease is becoming resistant even to the newest and best of the antibiotics. Without treatment, about 30 percent of patients die.

Humans shed the bacteria in their stool, which then contaminates water or food. Susceptible persons later consume the contaminated water or food. The spread of this disease directly from one person to another is uncommon.

Two to 5 percent of untreated typhoid fever patients shed the bacteria in their stool for years and years and so, like "Typhoid Mary," they become a source of infection for many other persons. They are called chronic carriers.

Typhoid fever is common on the Indian subcontinent and in developing countries in Latin America, Asia, and Africa. Worldwide, an estimated 16 million cases and 600,000 deaths are reported each year from typhoid fever. About 1.3 out of 500,000 U.S. citizens got typhoid fever while traveling abroad in the early 1990s.

### How effective is typhoid vaccine, and who should get it?

There are three different typhoid vaccines: one is given by mouth (Ty21a) and two are injected (the ViCPS, or "Vi" form, and an older inactivated form). Each protects roughly 50 to 80 percent of recipients. The schedule depends on the age of the recipient and on the form used. The vaccine given by mouth requires careful adherence to a somewhat complex eight-day regimen. The "Vi" form requires one injection initially. The other injected form initially requires two doses separated by at least four weeks (see Table 20-1).

No country currently requires typhoid fever vaccine for entry. However, because there is a risk of typhoid fever for U.S. travelers, the vaccine is recommended for those who will have prolonged exposure to potentially contaminated food and drink while visiting the Indian subcontinent, or developing countries in Latin America, Asia, or Africa. Vaccination is of particular value for persons who will be visiting smaller cities, villages, and rural areas.

Vaccination should not be used as a substitute for careful avoidance of contaminated food and beverages.

## Who should *not* get the vaccine?

✛ Persons with a history of a severe allergic or systemic reaction following a prior dose of typhoid fever vaccine or any of its components should not receive the vaccine.

✛ Persons with a moderate or severe acute illness should postpone vaccination.

✛ Persons with typhoid fever or who are chronic carriers of it should not receive the vaccine.

✛ A pregnant woman should receive the typhoid fever vaccine only if it is clearly needed.

### Injected typhoid vaccines

✛ The ViCPS form is not recommended for children less than 2 years old. The older inactivated form of the vaccine is effective for children as young as 6 months old.

### Oral typhoid vaccine

✛ Children less than 6 years old should not receive the vaccine.

✛ Persons who are immuno-compromised should not take this vaccine.

✠ Persons with fever, persistent diarrhea, or vomiting should not receive this vaccine.

✠ Persons who are on medications to kill bacteria, viruses, or malaria should discuss this vaccine with their healthcare provider before receiving it. Vaccination may need to be postponed.

## What are the vaccine risks and side effects?

### Injected typhoid vaccines

✠ Tenderness, swelling, and redness at the typhoid fever vaccine injection site commonly start within 6 to 24 hours and last a day or two.

✠ About half as many persons experience generalized symptoms after the Vi form than after the older vaccine. After the older vaccine, fever, muscle aches, and nausea each effect a few percent of recipients and about 10 percent get a headache.

✠ Severe allergic reactions and other severe reactions occur rarely after either injected typhoid fever vaccine.

### Oral typhoid vaccine

Although side effects may occur, they usually resolve on their own without medical care. Side effects may include hives or problems with the digestive tract (nausea, vomiting, diarrhea, abdominal cramps).

**Table 20-1**

## ADVANTAGES AND DISADVANTAGES OF THE THREE TYPHOID VACCINES

| VACCINE TYPE | ROUTE | SCHEDULE | SIDE EFFECTS | YOUNGEST AGE |
|---|---|---|---|---|
| Ty21a (Oral Typhoid) | by mouth | complicated regimen over 8 days | nausea, vomiting<br>fever: 0–5%<br>headache: 0–5% | 6 years |
| ViCPS | injected | 1 dose initially | injection site reactions, small: 7%<br>fever: 0–1%<br>headache: 2–3% | 2 years |
| Parenteral inactivated (older) | injected | 2 doses separated by 4 weeks | injection site reaction, severe: 3–35%<br>fever: 7–24%<br>headache: 9–10% | 6 months |

*Source: Based on* Health Information for International Travel, 1999–2000, *CDC*

## Additional notes

Plague vaccine and cholera vaccine often cause side effects much as the older injected typhoid fever vaccine does. Theoretically, getting these vaccines at the same time could lead to a bigger reaction. If you have time to separate these vaccinations by a week or more and still get all the vaccines you need before travel, you may have less discomfort.

## YELLOW FEVER

### What is yellow fever, how is it spread, and how is it treated?

Epidemics of yellow fever were recorded as long ago as 1648. The yellow fever virus, a member of the *flaviviridae* (*flavus*, L. "yellow"), is spread by the *Aedes aeypti* mosquito, as demonstrated by Dr. Walter Reed in 1900. Two researchers at the Rockefeller Foundation in New York developed a vaccine that was tested in human volunteers in 1936 and found it to be effective. Indeed, the vaccine, along with mosquito control measures, were so effective that by the end of World War II yellow fever was considered a medical curiosity. In the early 1980s about 200 cases were reported annually to the World Health Organization from the African continent, but by the late 1980s as many as 5,000 cases were reported from this region in a single year. Because the yellow fever is easily mistaken for other diseases, it is likely that only a small fraction of the actual cases are reported.

Although the mosquitoes that spread the virus live in many warm climates, yellow fever occurs only in sub-Saharan Africa and the northern half of South America (see Figure 20-3). Unlike the rural mosquitoes that spread Japanese encephalitis, the yellow fever mosquitoes live in the city or the jungle.

Most persons infected with the yellow fever virus have no symptoms, but those who develop symptoms begin to do so within three to six days of the mosquito bite. Symptoms include headache, fever, photophobia (extreme sensitivity to and fear of light), pain in the lower spine and extremities, loss of appetite, upper abdominal tenderness, and vomiting.

As many as 15 percent of persons who become infected develop moderate or life-threatening symptoms: jaundice (liver distress that causes yellowing of the skin and eyes—hence the name "yellow fever"), bloody vomit and stools, decreased urine (a sign of kidney distress), and coma. The only treatment is

**Figure 20-3**
## YELLOW FEVER ZONES IN SOUTH AMERICA AND AFRICA

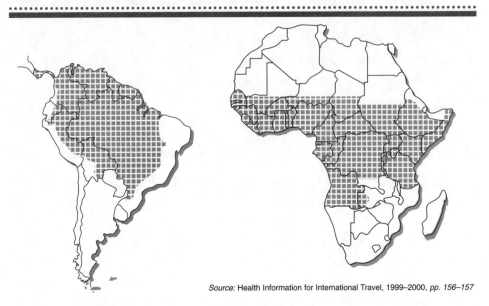

*Source:* Health Information for International Travel, 1999–2000, *pp. 156–157*

supportive care. Many of the persons with severe yellow fever do not recover. In Africa between 1986 and 1995, 24 percent of those who contracted yellow fever died from it.

To minimize your risk of mosquito bites, follow these tips: The urban mosquitoes that spread yellow fever primarily feed during the day, so stay in air-conditioned or well-screened quarters. If you go outside, wear a long-sleeved shirt and long pants and apply an insect repellent containing perme-thrin to your clothes. Wear mosquito repellent containing DEET on exposed skin. In rural areas, sleep under permethrin-impregnated mosquito netting or in a screened room. Also use insecticidal space sprays.

### How effective is yellow fever vaccine, and who should get it?

A single dose begins to protect the recipient in 7 to 10 days. A booster is recommended subsequently every 10 years if exposure persists. The vaccine is effective in essentially all recipients.

Some countries require proof of yellow fever vaccination on an International Certificate of Vaccination (or an official letter of exemption) whether you are traveling to them or just passing through them. At least 10 days prior to arrival, the vaccine must be administered at an approved Yellow Fever Vaccination Center. Contact your state or local health department to locate such a center in your area and to learn the most current requirements.

Irrespective of border requirements, the vaccine is recommended for persons living or traveling in yellow fever–infected areas. This includes urban and non-urban areas where yellow fever actually is being reported, and non-urban areas anywhere within the yellow fever zone (sub-Saharan African and the northern part of South America).

## Who should *not* get the vaccine?

⊕ Persons with a history of a severe allergic or systemic reaction following a prior dose of yellow fever vaccine or any of its components (such as eggs) should not take yellow fever vaccine. There are no antibiotics or preservatives in the vaccine.

⊕ Persons who have a moderate or severe acute illness should postpone vaccination.

⊕ The American Academy of Pediatrics states that yellow fever vaccine should not be given to children less than 4 months old and that the decision to give it to children 4 to 9 months old should be based upon the risk of disease exposure.

⊕ Pregnant women should only receive this vaccine if travel to a high-risk area is unavoidable.

⊕ The ACIP recommends that immuno-compromised patients who cannot avoid travel to yellow fever–infected areas should be advised of the risk, informed on how to avoid the mosquitoes that spread the disease, and given a waiver.

## What are the vaccine risks and side effects?

The results of studies done on the side effects of yellow fever vary a lot. In general, few persons develop side effects, and when they do the reactions are mild (such as pain and redness at the injection site shortly after vaccination or fever, mild headache, or muscle aches about a week after vaccination), and these side effects do not last long. Severe allergic reactions and other severe reactions occur rarely (fewer than 1 out of 1 million persons). The persons affected are usually allergic to eggs or are younger than 9 months old.

## CONCLUSION

While formal vaccination requirements for leaving the United States no longer exist, specialized vaccines may be required by the country you are visiting and it is important to be aware of these. Irrespective of national requirements, you may want to receive vaccines that offer protection from diseases to which you and your family could be exposed. It is especially important to protect traveling children since they are at greater risk of exposure to certain contagious diseases because they are less likely to be careful about avoiding germs.

Of course, you will have other health considerations in addition to vaccines. For example, medication may be necessary to protect you and your family from diseases such as malaria and travelers' diarrhea. Such preparations should be made in consultation with a knowledgeable person and a good travel health guide.

The better prepared you are, the more fun you're likely to have when you arrive at your destination. Have a great trip!

*The scars of others should teach us caution.*

—St. Jerome

# Chapter 21

# Vaccines and Bioterrorism:
## Smallpox and Anthrax

The fear that biologic agents could be used in acts of aggression against a population is expressed in a single word: bioterrorism. The relative ease and economy of turning germs into weapons may appeal to rogue nations and terrorist groups.

Though many infectious diseases could be used by terrorists, we will focus on two diseases that should have been of little concern to twenty-first century parents: anthrax, the fifth of the biblical plagues (1491 BC), which in recent times has affected only about 2000 persons worldwide per year; and smallpox, which was already painstakingly eradicated once from the globe.

These two diseases may be prevented through vaccination, and very frequently citizens ask the CDC to provide them with the vaccines. Anthrax and smallpox vaccines are neither recommended for, nor available to, the general public. Just as frequently, parents question the CDC about the safety and effectiveness of the anthrax vaccine because it is required for many military personnel and because some believe it was a cause of Gulf War syndrome. We have included this chapter so you can understand the diseases and vaccines that you are hearing about in the news.

# SMALLPOX

In 1979 physicians stopped giving the smallpox vaccine after the disease was officially eradicated from the globe. However, the United States still has live smallpox virus under lock and key at the CDC in Atlanta, Georgia—just in case the U.S. ever needs to mass-produce the smallpox vaccine again in response to a threat of germ warfare.

Smallpox was highly contagious—as contagious as chickenpox, but a tad less than measles—and easily spread within a household. Usually, smallpox infection occurred when a person inhaled droplets of mucus discharged from the nose, mouth, or throat of someone with the smallpox rash (see Figure 22-1). The blisters also contained infected material, so handling the laundry of a smallpox patient could be dangerous. One account describes smallpox as spreading in 14-day waves, with each wave from 10 to 20 times as large as the last.

Smallpox may have emerged as a human disease as much as 12,000 years ago. The effects of smallpox have been found on Egyptian mummies from 1580 to 1350 BC, and relics of smallpox gods have been found in India, China, and parts of Africa. By the end of the eighteenth century in Europe, about 400,000 people died of smallpox each year.

When European explorers inadvertently imported smallpox to the Americas, the disease decimated the Aztec and Incan empires. Later, smallpox was used deliberately as a biologic weapon against Native Americans; Europeans wiped out entire tribes by giving smallpox patients' blankets to unsuspecting Native Americans.

For centuries, people were able to obtain some protection by taking dried scabs of the pox from smallpox victims and inhaling or inoculating the material. Unfortunately, although these persons' bouts with smallpox

**Figure 22-1**
**SMALLPOX**

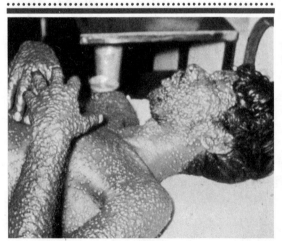

Source: CDC

may have been milder, they still spread the disease to others. A huge breakthrough came in 1796, when Edward Jenner discovered that inoculating people with cowpox protected them against the smallpox disease.

Less than two hundred years later, on May 8, 1980, the World Health Organization certified that smallpox had been eradicated from the planet. Vaccination was no longer necessary.

Governments and epidemiologists debated whether the laboratory specimens of smallpox virus should also be destroyed, so no one would accidentally or intentionally release the virus on a population that was no longer immune. The two-hundredth anniversary of Jenner's discovery, 1996, was set as the date to destroy the remaining virus—some in a Russian lab, some at the CDC in Atlanta. U.S. President Bill Clinton decided that what was left of the virus in the U.S. should not be destroyed, just in case Americans ever needed to be vaccinated again for the explosively contagious, deadly disease.

The threat of smallpox being used in biowarfare is considered "low probability, high impact," according to Dean Mason of the CDC. He says the United States has been considering stockpiling smallpox for the development of a vaccine in this country. We "don't want to be alarmist," he explains, "but we do want to be proactive." He continues that the likelihood of smallpox being used as bioterrorism is "remote."

## ANTHRAX

Though in the 1950s an estimated 20,000 to 100,000 cases of anthrax occurred in the world each year, by the 1990s only around 2,000 cases occurred annually.

### What is anthrax?

Anthrax is a spore-forming bacterium found in the soil throughout the world. The spores are so resistant to environmental conditions that they may survive in soil for 25 years—or possibly as long as a century. The spores cause a common disease among grazing animals, such as cows and sheep, and humans are usually infected via animal products, so vaccination of these animals in the U.S. is the rule. Infection manifests in three different disease forms, depending on which part of the body was primarily infected:

the skin, the digestive system, or the lungs. The lethality of the disease also depends on its primary location: fewer than 5 percent of patients die from anthrax of the skin, 25 to 75 percent die from the digestive tract variety, and almost 100 percent die if the anthrax spores are inhaled into the lungs.

Antibiotics can be used after exposure to anthrax, but they must be used prior to the onset of symptoms, and treatment should include vaccination. Almost all cases of inhalational anthrax have resulted in death, even with post-exposure treatment.

## What is the anthrax vaccine?

In 1970, an anthrax vaccine became fully licensed for use in humans. It does not contain live cells, unlike the vaccine used in animals. The vaccine is not licensed for use in children or pregnant women.

After the first dose of anthrax vaccine, additional doses are given 2 and 4 weeks later, and again 6, 12, and 18 months after the first. Boosters are given each year thereafter if exposure (or the risk of exposure) continues.

The vaccine is almost 93 percent effective at preventing the occurrence of skin anthrax in adults. No data on its effectiveness in children are available. Although there are too few cases of lung anthrax to test the vaccine's effectiveness against this form, which is most lethal, some studies with experimental monkeys indicate effectiveness. Because the duration of protection has not been established, boosters are recommended if exposure or risk is continued.

## Who should and should *not* get the vaccine?

People who are at significant, continuing risk of acquiring anthrax should receive the vaccine. This includes some military personnel, as well as individuals with industrial, agricultural, or laboratory exposure to anthrax.

This vaccine, which has been required for some military personnel, has become quite controversial. Top military officials have said the vaccine is absolutely necessary to protect service personnel against hostile nations that have the capability of using deadly biologic agents in such places as the Persian Gulf region. Nevertheless, many military personnel concerned about adverse side effects have refused to receive the vaccine.

Anthrax vaccine should *not* be given to anyone with a hypersensitivity reaction to the vaccine. People who actually had anthrax in the past should not be vaccinated because they may develop severe symptoms at the site of injection.

## What are the vaccine risks and side effects?

Reactions such as redness and tenderness within a day and lasting a day or two are not much more frequent than they are after the injection of sterile saltwater. Very rarely, swelling extends from the shoulder to the forearm. Also rare is the development of a painless nodule that lasts for up to three weeks at the site of injection. About 7 per 1,000 vaccine recipients get a slight headache or muscle aches, or simply do not feel well for a day or two. An estimated 5 out of 100,000 vaccine recipients will have a more significant reaction. For example, from 1990 to 1999 two cases of Guillain-Barré syndrome were reported to the Vaccine Adverse Event Reporting System after anthrax vaccine. But researchers do not know if the GBS was caused by the vaccine.

*It is difficult to say what is impossible, for the dream of yesterday is the hope of today and the reality of tomorrow.*

—Robert H. Goddard

# Chapter 22

# Future Vaccines

Dozens of innovative vaccines are currently undergoing testing or awaiting approval by the U.S. Food and Drug Administration. It's conceivable that one day in the future, vaccines will ward off dozens of additional diseases, both infectious and noninfectious (such as cancer). Advances in molecular biology and genetic research hold the promise of huge health benefits.

## Nasal Spray Flu Vaccine

If you hate having your child get a flu shot, a new prescription nasal spray may be just what the doctor will order. The spray flu vaccine, called FluMist, was developed by Aviron. The company has completed a trial that proved the spray 93 percent effective against influenza and 98 percent effective against ear infection, a common complication of the flu in children. (More details are provided in Chapter 16.) This vaccine may be approved for pediatric use by 2002.

## Respiratory Syncytial Virus (RSV) Vaccine

RSV causes respiratory infections in infants and toddlers, often developing into pneumonia and bronchitis in children less than a year old. In newborns it can cause irritability, poor feeding, and episodes when the infant stops breathing. An infant who was born prematurely or has a congenital heart defect, lung disease, or a weakened immune system is at risk for having a severe case of RSV. Some children infected with RSV develop chronic wheezing. Currently, concentrated RSV antibodies are given to infants with severe RSV, but a vaccine would prevent thousands of emergency visits and hospital stays. RSV vaccine is still being tested and may be available by 2005.

## Rotavirus Vaccine

Rotavirus causes diarrhea. It is so easily spread in stool that we almost all have been infected by the time we are 5 years old, and most people get rotavirus more than once. The first bout is the worst, causing dehydration and body salt imbalances, which may require intravenous fluids. In the U.S., rotavirus is responsible for more than 500,000 visits to physicians' offices and emergency departments, more than 50,000 hospitalizations, and 10 to 40 deaths each year. Among infants and young children throughout the world, rotavirus is the leading cause of severely dehydrating diarrhea, killing 1,600 to 2,400 each day.

The first rotavirus vaccine was licensed in the U.S. in August 1998, but was withdrawn from the market when it was shown to cause a form of bowel obstruction. The vaccine was given by mouth and contained live viruses, much like the wild rotavirus virus, but weakened.

Other rotavirus vaccines are in development for use in the U.S., but extensive testing will be necessary to demonstrate their safety. It is unlikely that another vaccine will be available here until between 2005 and 2010. Until then, parents should realize that rotavirus diarrhea can be severe. If caught early, most cases can be managed using small, frequent feedings of fluids specially designed for rehydration; in severe cases intravenous fluids may be needed. It is important not to allow infants or young children to become dehydrated and not to replace diarrhea, which is full of body salts, with plain water.

## MALARIA VACCINE

Although malaria is almost unheard of in the U.S., worldwide it is the single leading cause of death in children younger than 5 years. Each year, an estimated 200 to 500 million persons are infected with malaria, and 1 million to 2.7 million persons die from it. The vast majority of these cases occur in young children in sub-Saharan Africa.

Ripley Ballou (formerly with Walter Reed Hospital and currently the Director of Clinical Development for the company Medimmune) says the U.S. Army has been working on a malaria vaccine since the 1970s. Malaria has been a major problem for soldiers dating back to the Revolutionary War. According to Ballou, it's "one of the highest priority infectious disease problems the Army has focused on." A vaccine is important, he explains, because human bodies do not easily tolerate preventive drugs, and worse yet, the parasites develop a resistance to the drugs "as fast as they're created." Ballou emphasizes that coming up with an effective vaccine is particularly difficult because malaria can re-infect a person over and over, even with the same strain. He says the disease, which has infected humans even "before we were human, knows more about our immune systems than we do." Malaria has some 6,000 genes and 14 chromosomes, more than some insects.

Still, he is optimistic that one day we will have a malaria vaccine. "Several vaccines are now in clinical trials," he explains. "The most promising are still years from licensure." They're being tested on persons in endemic countries. Ballou has been personally involved in 20 different trials with human volunteers; in fact, he tested his first vaccine on himself. (It did not work, and he ended up with malaria.)

## TUBERCULOSIS (TB) VACCINE

One out of three people in the world is infected with the tuberculosis bacterium, and 4 billion people have received the vaccine. The current vaccine, BCG, is effective against severe complications of TB in children, but it does little to protect against tuberculosis of the lungs in adults. (See Chapter 19 for details.)

Thanks to developments in microbiology, genetics, and biotechnology, there is hope for a new and improved tuberculosis vaccine in the foreseeable future, according to the World Health Organization.

## AIDS Vaccine

HIV (human immunodeficiency virus) is the virus responsible for AIDS, the acquired immunodeficiency syndrome first identified in 1981. Worldwide by the end of 1997, 30 million persons were infected with HIV, and experts suspected the toll would climb to 40 million by 2000.

Because of the global epidemic, scientists in many countries are working to develop a vaccine, but their attempts have been hampered by the nature of the virus. For example, for most vaccines, scientists isolate the viral proteins that ignite our immune systems—but HIV proteins keep changing.

An HIV vaccine may be developed that does not prevent disease but at least slows the disease progression or reduces transmission to others. Though a vaccine that would successfully accomplish any of these would be welcome, experts do not anticipate that it will be available soon.

## Cytomegalic Virus (CMV) Vaccine

CMV is a virus that most people are exposed to and that usually causes minor respiratory illness, a form of infectious mononucleosis, or no symptoms at all. However, like rubella, CMV infection during the early months of pregnancy can cause damage to the developing fetus. Indeed, 10 to 15 percent of the infected fetuses will suffer permanent damage.

Transplant patients who were not previously infected with CMV but who receive a CMV-infected organ can also develop severe, even life-threatening illness. (And it can be difficult to find an organ donor who has never been infected with CMV.) Similarly, CMV often causes a deadly pneumonia in persons undergoing bone marrow transplants. Researchers are optimistic that eventually a CMV vaccine will be available to protect females before childbearing and potential transplant patients who were not previously infected.

## Ulcer Vaccine

A new vaccine promises to prevent many of the 22 million ulcer cases caused each year by the *Helicobacter pylori* bacterium. A preliminary study showed that all of the subjects who received the vaccine developed antibodies to *H. pylori,* whereas none of those who received the placebo developed them. Further studies are being conducted.

## CANCER VACCINES

Vaccines to slow cancers in the earliest stages are expected in the next few years. Several melanoma vaccines are in the final stages of clinical testing; safety trials are underway for vaccines against prostate and lung cancer. Still other studies hold promise in the fight against colon, stomach, cervical, and other cancers.

Scientists are working on vaccines that rev up the immune system to enable the body to reduce the size of tumors and even destroy cancerous cells. More than a dozen known antigens produced by breast, ovarian, lung, and prostate tumors are being looked at for potential vaccines.

Scientists have identified the immune cell capable of protecting women from breast and ovarian cancer, and this discovery will hasten development of a preventive vaccine.

But vaccines to *prevent* any form of cancer in healthy persons are not expected for more than a decade.

## ALZHEIMERS VACCINE

Alzheimers afflicts 4 million Americans: 1 out of 10 persons over age 65 and nearly half of those over 85. After two decades of research, a California biotech company is reporting promising initial results with a vaccine that might someday be used to treat Alzheimers disease. Working with mice, company scientists showed that they could prevent the buildup of a protein that characterizes the human disease. Researchers showed that—in mice, at least—an experimental vaccine can prevent and even reverse some of the brain lesions that are hallmarks of Alzheimers. It remains to be seen whether the vaccine will prove effective and safe for humans.

## PAINLESS VACCINES

In addition to new vaccines, new vaccine delivery systems are being developed that promise protection from disease without the painful prick of a needle. One day in the not too distant future, vaccines may be available in the form of a mouthwash, a time-released pill, genetically engineered food, or even a skin patch. Twelve billion skin injections are administered each year, according to the World Health Organization. Efforts to develop needle-free technology have intensified due to the risk of contamination from tainted needles coupled with the growing number of required vaccines, according to Bruce Weniger, Chief of Vaccine Development for the National Immunization Program. New vaccine delivery systems now being tested would not only eliminate painful local side effects that come with skin injection, but also reduce the risk of contamination and make it easier to store, transport, and administer vaccines.

## CONCLUSION

The future holds the exciting promise of safer and more easily administered formulations of current vaccines, as well as new vaccines for diseases that were not previously preventable. Remarkable progress in science is making these advances possible.

*The man who graduates today and stops learning tomorrow is uneducated the day after. But desire of knowledge, like the thirst of riches, increases ever with the acquisition.*

—Lawrence Stern

# Chapter 23

# Where to Learn More:
## Government Sources, Healthcare and Parent Organizations, and Pharmaceutical Companies

Here are addresses, telephone numbers, and Internet web sites you can use to find more information on vaccines. The following organizations are included for your reference only. *The opinions and data offered by these sources may vary in content and accuracy.*

## U.S. GOVERNMENT SOURCES

**Centers for Disease Control and Prevention (CDC),** National Immunization Program. This federal agency answers immunization questions from the public as well as from healthcare professionals.

    1600 Clifton Road, NE, MS E-05

    Atlanta, GA 30333

Vaccine Hotline: To speak with information specialists for the CDC Monday through Friday, 8 A.M. to 11 P.M., Eastern Time, call

    800-232-2522 (English)

    800-232-0233 (Spanish)

Immunization Information: 800-CDC-SHOT (an automated information service)

National Immunization Program: www.cdc.gov/nip

See especially the childhood immunization schedule, the adult schedule, the
  ACIP index, the Vaccine Safety homepage, as well as the vaccine
  information statements.
CDC's weekly reports about diseases in *Morbidity & Mortality Weekly
  Reports (MMWR)*: www.cdc.gov/epo/mmwr
> Travel health information: www.cdc.gov/travel/index.htm
> National Center for Infectious Diseases: www.cdc.gov/ncidod
> CDC Fax Back System for immunization information:
> 888-232-3299.

**Vaccine Adverse Event Reporting System (VAERS)** is a reporting system created by the FDA and the CDC to receive and analyze reports about negative side effects that may be associated with vaccines. VAERS encourages
reporting of significant side effects after vaccination. A report does not confirm that a vaccine caused the problem and does not enter a person into the
vaccine injury compensation process.

> P.O. Box 1100
> Rockville, MD 20849-1100
> Phone: (800) 822-7967 (24 hours a day)
> Web site: www.fda.gov/cber/vaers/vaers.htm or www.cdc.gov/nip/vaers.htm
> E-mail: vaers@cber.fda.gov or VAERS@cais.com

**Food and Drug Administration (FDA).** Under the National Childhood
Vaccine Injury Act of 1986, consumers are entitled to information on reports
about side effects after vaccination. This is the group to contact if you'd like
access to such information.

> 5600 Fishers Lane
> Rockville, MD 20857
> Phone: (888) 463-6332
> Fax: (301) 443-1726
> Web site: www.fda.gov

**National Vaccine Injury Compensation Program (NVICP).** Congress passed
the National Childhood Vaccine Injury Act in an effort to ensure vaccine

safety and to compensate people injured by vaccines. NVICP can give you information on how to file a claim, the criteria for eligibility, and the documentation required.

> Parklawn Building, Room 8A-46
> 5600 Fishers Lane
> Rockville, MD 20857
> Phone: (800) 338-2382 or (301) 443-8196
> Fax: (301) 443-8196
> Web site: www.hrsa.gov/bhpr/vicp

**Healthcare Financing Administration.** This federal agency provides information on Medicare (adult immunization), Medicaid, and the Child Health insurance programs.

> Web site: www.hcfa.gov

**National Institutes of Health,** National Institute of Allergy and Infectious Diseases.

> Web site: www.niaid.nih.gov/publications

**Department of Defense,** information on anthrax.

> Web site: www.anthrax.osd.mil

## HEALTHCARE ORGANIZATIONS

**American Academy of Pediatrics (AAP).** Forty-five thousand pediatricians focus on the health, safety, and well-being of American children.

> 141 Northwest Point Boulevard
> Elk Grove Village, IL 60007-1098
> Phone: (800) 433-9016
> Fax: (847) 228-5097
> Web site: www.aap.org
> E-mail: kidsdocs@aap.org

**American Pharmaceutical Association (APhA).** This group of some 50,000 pharmacists and health professionals attempts to educate the public about pharmaceutical products, including vaccines.

2215 Constitution Avenue, NW
Washington, DC 20037-2985
Phone: (202) 628-4410
Fax: (202) 783-2351
Web site: www.aphanet.org

**Every Child By Two (ECBT)**, set up by the American Nurses Foundation, works
to raise awareness of the need for timely immunization of children by age 2.
666 11th St., NW, Suite 202
Washington, DC 20001
Phone: (202) 783-7035
Web site: www.ecbt.org
E-mail: info@ecbt.org

**Immunization Action Coalition (IAC)** is a nonprofit group that attempts to
boost immunization rates. Their free publication, called NEEDLE TIPS, a
28-page semiannual publication usually used by healthcare professionals,
has some useful information. Parents may be especially interested in the
vaccine information statements, the disease photos, and "Ask the Experts."
1573 Selby Avenue
Saint Paul, MN 55104
Phone: (651) 647-9009
Fax: (651) 647-9131
Web site: www.immunize.org
E-mail: admin@immunize.org

**Infectious Disease Society of America (IDSA)** provides information on dis-
ease prevention to the public and healthcare providers.
99 Canal Center Plaza, Suite 210
Alexandria, VA 22314
Phone: (703) 299-0200
Fax: (703) 299-0204
Web site: www.idsociety.org; www.immunizationinfo.org
E-mail: info@idsociety.org

**Institute for Vaccine Safety** distributes information on vaccine recommendations, investigates safety concerns, and funds relevant research projects.

> Johns Hopkins School of Public Health
> 615 North Wolfe Street, Suite W5515
> Baltimore, MD 21207
> Phone: (410) 955-2955
> Fax: (410) 502-6733
> Web site: www.vaccinesafety.edu
> E-mail: info@vaccinesafety.edu

**World Health Organization (WHO),** Department of Vaccines and Other Biologicals, was established by WHO to protect those at risk against vaccine-preventable diseases. It focuses on immunization programs, vaccine research and development, and vaccine supply and quality.

> Avenue Appia 20 1211
> Geneva 27, Switzerland
> Phone: (+41 22) 791 2111
> Fax: (+41 22) 791 0746
> Web site: www.who.int/gpv or www.who.int/gpv-safety
> E-mail: info@who.ch

**American College Health Association** provides information on vaccines for college students, especially the meningococcus vaccine.

> Web site: www.acha.org

**National Coalition for Adult Immunization.**

> Web site: www.nfid.org/ncai

**ImmunoFacts' Immunization Gateway,** a service to medical offices, provides links to state, national, and international vaccine information programs.

> Web site: www.immunofacts.com

## Parent Groups

**Parents of Kids with Infectious Diseases (PKIDs)** offers parents information about infectious diseases.

    P.O. Box 5666
    Vancouver, WA 98668
    Phone: (877) 55P-KIDS or (360) 695-0293
    Web site: www.pkids.org
    E-mail: pkids@pkids.org

**Informed Parents against VAPP** consists of parents who have long fought the use of oral polio vaccine due to Vaccine Associated Paralytic Polio.

    P.O. Box 53212
    Washington, DC 20009
    Phone: (888) 363-8277
    Web site: www.ipav.org

**Vaccine Information & Awareness (VIA)** empowers parents to challenge, research, and become more informed about vaccine risks. The site is operated by one person, Karin Schumacher.

    Phone: 619-339-5498
    E-mail via@access1.net
    Web site: www.access1.net/via

**National Vaccine Information Center (NVIC)**, also maintained by Karin Schumacher, was created by a mom whose son had a severe reaction after a vaccination. The NVIC warns parents about problems that might occur and assists parents whose children have health problems believed to have been caused by vaccination.

    512 West Maple Ave, Suite 206
    Vienna, VA 22180
    Phone: (800) 909-SHOT
    E-mail: info@909shot.com
    Web site: www.909shot.com

# PHARMACEUTICAL MANUFACTURERS AND DISTRIBUTORS

Aventis Pasteur
P.O. Box 187, Discovery Drive
Swiftwater, PA 18370
Phone: (800) 822-2463 or (570) 839-7187
Web site: http://209.37.191.29/

Merck & Co., Inc.
Merck Vaccine Division
Bldg. 97 / P.O. Box 4
West Point, PA 19486-0004
Phone: (800) NSC MERCK
Web site: www.VaccinesbyNet.com

North American Vaccine, Inc.
12103 Indian Creek Ct.
Beltsville, MD 20745
Phone: (301) 470-6100
Web site: www.nava.com

SmithKline Beecham
1 Franklin Place
P.O. Box 7929
Philadelphia, PA 19101-7929
Phone: (800) 366-8900 or (215) 751-4912
Web site: www.sb.com

Wyeth-Lederle Vaccines and Pediatrics
Five Giralda Farms
American Home Products Corp.
Madison, NJ 07940
Phone: (201) 660-5000
Web site: www.ahp.com

# References

All quoted material, unless indicated otherwise, comes from personal interviews between Cynthia Good and the persons named.

## GENERAL REFERENCES

Atkinson, W., S. Humiston, S. Wolfe, and R. Nelson, eds. 1999. *Epidemiology and Prevention of Vaccine-Preventable Diseases.* 5th ed. Atlanta: U.S. Department of Health and Human Services (DHHS), Centers for Disease Control and Prevention (CDC). For a copy, call (800) 41-TRAIN.

CDC. 1998. *State Immunization Requirements, 1998–1999.* Atlanta: DHHS.

———. 1999. *Health Information for International Travel, 1999–2000.* Atlanta: DHHS. For a copy, call (202) 512-1800.

———. Weekly. *Morbidity and Mortality Weekly Report (MMWR).* Published by the Epidemiology Program Office. Atlanta: DHHS. See http://www2.cdc.gov/mmwr for online issues.

———. Ongoing. *Recommendations of the Advisory Committee on Immunization Practices (ACIP).* Atlanta: DHHS. These are usually printed in *MMWR.* See specific references.

Evans, A. S., and R. A. Kaslow, eds. 1997. *Viral Infections in Humans: Epidemiology and Control.* 4th ed. New York: Plenum.

Grabenstein, J. D., and L. A. Grabenstein. 1997. *Pocket Immunofacts™ Vaccines and Immunologics.* Norwell, MA: Kluwer, Facts and Comparisons.

Immunization Action Coalition. *Needle Tips* and the *Hepatitis B Coalition News.* See also http://www.immunize.org for online versions of these periodicals.

Peter, G., ed. 1997. *1997 Red Book: Report of the Committee on Infectious Diseases.* 24th ed. Elk Grove Village, IL: American Academy of Pediatrics.

Plotkin, S. A., and W. A. Orenstein, eds. 1999. *Vaccines.* 3rd ed. Philadelphia: Harcourt, Saunders.

Rose, S. R. 1999. *International Travel HealthGuide.* 10th ed. Northampton, MA: Travel Medicine.

Stratton, K. R., C. J. Howe, and R. B. Johnston, Jr., eds. 1994. *Adverse Events Associated with Childhood Vaccines: Evidence Bearing on Causality.* Vaccine Safety Committee, Division of Health Promotion and Disease Prevention, Institute of Medicine. Washington: National Academy Press.

## SPECIFIC REFERENCES

**Chapter 4: How Vaccines Get Recommended**

CDC. 1999. Intussusception among recipients of rotavirus vaccine: United States, 1998–1999. *MMWR* 48, no. 27: 577-581.

———. 1999. Rotavirus vaccine for the prevention of rotavirus gastroenteritis among children: Recommendations of the ACIP. *MMWR* 48, no. RR-2.

Orenstein, W. A., and A. R. Hinman. 1999. The immunization system in the United States: The role of school immunization laws. *Vaccine* 17 (supplement): S19–S24.

**Chapter 5: Vaccine Controversies**

Autism Working Group. 1996. State of the science in autism: Report to the National Institutes of Health. *Journal of Autism and Developmental Disorders* 26, no. 2: 121–54.

Classen, D. C., and J. Classen. 1997. The timing of pediatric immunization and the risk of insulin-dependent diabetes mellitus. *Infectious Diseases in Clinical Practice* 6: 449–54.

Ellenberg, Susan S. 1999. (Director, Biostatistics and Epidemiology Division, Center for Biologics Evaluation and Research, U.S. Federal Drug Administration). Testimony before the U.S. House of Representatives Committee on Government Reform, Subcommittee on Criminal Justice, Drug Policy, and Human Resources (May 18).

Graves P. M., K. J. Barriga, J. M. Norris, et al. 1999. Lack of association between early childhood immunizations and beta-cell autoimmunity. Diabetes Care 22, no. 10: 1694–97.

Halsey, Neal. 1999. Testimony before the U.S. House of Representatives Committee on Government Reform (October 12).

Henderson, J., K. North, M. Griffiths, et al. 1999. Pertussis vaccination and wheezing illnesses in young children: Prospective cohort study. The longitudinal study of pregnancy and childhood team. *BMJ* 318, no. 7192 (May 18): 1173–76.

Margolis, Harold. 1999. (Chief, Hepatitis Branch, Division of Viral and Rickettsial Diseases, National Center for Infectious Diseases, CDC). Testimony before the U.S. House of Representatives Committee on Government Reform, Subcommittee on Criminal Justice, Drug Policy, and Human Resources (May 18).

Taylor, B., E. Miller, C. P. Farrington, et al. 1999. Autism and measles, mumps, and rubella vaccine: No epidemiological evidence for a causal association. *Lancet* 353 (June): 2026–29.

**Chapter 7: Parents' Rights**

Bowen, Jon. 1999. Disease parties. *Health and Body,* 26 October.

*Dalli v. Board of Education.* 1971. 358 Mass. 753.

Ehresmann, K. R., C. W. Hedberg, M. B. Grimm, et al. 1995. An outbreak of measles at an international sporting event with airborne transmission in a domed stadium. *Journal of Infectious Diseases* 171, no. 3: 679–83.

Gellen, B., E. Maibach, and E. K. Marcuse. 1999. National Network for Immunization Information. Unpublished data.

Newsweek. 1999. Vaccines: Are they worth it? *Newsweek* 13 September.

Orenstein, W. A., and A. R. Hinman. 1999. The immunization system in the United States: The role of school immunization laws. *Vaccine 17* (supplement): S19–S24.

Salmon, D. A., et al. 1999. Health consequences of religious and philosophical exemptions from immunization laws: Individual and societal risk of measles. *Journal of the American Medical Association,* 282, no. 1: 47–53.

**Chapter 8: Hepatitis B Vaccine**

ACIP. 1999 update. Hepatitis B virus infection: A comprehensive immunization strategy to eliminate transmission in the United States. Recommendations of the ACIP. Draft distributed for public comment at the open meeting of ACIP in Atlanta (June 8).

Grotto, I., Y. Mandel, M. Ephrost, et al. 1998. Major adverse reactions to yeast-derived hepatitis B vaccine: A review. *Vaccine* 16: 329–34.

Margolis, Harold. 1999. (Chief, Hepatitis Branch, Division of Viral and Rickettsial Diseases, National Center for Infectious Diseases, CDC). Testimony before the U.S. House of Representatives Committee on Government Reform, Subcommittee on Criminal Justice, Drug Policy, and Human Resources (May 18).

Mast, E., F. J. Mahoney, M. J. Alter, and H. S. Margolis. 1998. Progress toward elimination of hepatitis B virus transmission in the United States. *Vaccine* 16 (supplement): S48–S51.

**Chapter 9: DTaP Vaccine: Diphtheria, Tetanus, and Acellular Pertussis**

ACIP. 1997. Pertussis vaccination: Use of acellular pertussis vaccines among infants and young children. Recommendations of the ACIP. *MMWR* 46, no. RR-7 (28 March): 1–25.

Ellenberg, Susan S. 1999. (Director, Biostatistics and Epidemiology Division, Center for Biologics Evaluation and Research, U.S. Federal Drug Administration). Testimony before the U.S. House of Representatives Committee on Government Reform, Subcommittee on Criminal Justice, Drug Policy, and Human Resources (May 18).

Scheifele, S., R. Halperin, and R. Pless. 1999. Marked reduction in febrile seizures and hypotonic-hyporesponsive episodes with acellular pertussis-based vaccines: Results of Canada-wide surveillance, 1993–1998. Abstract presented at the Annual Meeting of the Infectious Disease Society of America (November).

**Chapter 10: Polio Vaccine**

ACIP. 1997. Poliomyelitis prevention in the United States: Introduction of a sequential vaccination schedule of inactivated poliovirus vaccine followed by oral poliovirus vaccine. Recommendations of the ACIP. *MMWR* 46, no. RR-3 (24 January): 1–25.

———. 1999. Progress toward the global interruption of wild poliovirus type 2 transmission. Recommendations of the ACIP. *MMWR* 48, no. 33 (27 August): 736–38, 747.

———. 1999. Revised recommendation for routine poliomyelitis vaccination: Recommendations of the ACIP. *MMWR* 48, no. 27 (16 July): 590.

Strebel, P.M., R. W. Sutter, S. L. Cochi, et al. 1992. Epidemiology of poliomyelitis in the United States one decade after the last reported case of indigenous wild virus-associated disease. *Clinical Infectious Diseases* 14 (February): 568–79.

**Chapter 11: Hib Vaccine**

ACIP. 1991. *Haemophilus* B conjugate vaccines for prevention of *Haemophilus influenzae* type B disease among infants and children two months of age and older. *MMWR* 40, no. RR-1 (11 January): 1–7.

———. 1998. Progress toward eliminating *Haemophilus influenzae* type B disease among infants and children: United States, 1987–1997. *MMWR* 47, no. 46 (27 November): 993–98.

## Chapter 12: MMR Vaccine

ACIP. 1998. Measles, mumps, and rubella: Vaccine use and strategies for elimination of measles, rubella, and congenital rubella syndrome and control of mumps. Recommendations of the ACIP. *MMWR* 47, no. RR-8 (22 May): 1–57.

CDC. 1996. *Six Common Misconceptions About Vaccination and How to Respond to Them.* Atlanta: DHHS.

———. 1999. Epidemiology of measles in the United States. *MMWR* 48, no. 34 (3 September): 749–53.

———. 1999. Measles update from the National Immunization Program. Weeks 37–41, no. 5 (22 October).

———. 1999. Rubella outbreak: Westchester County, New York, 1997–1998. *MMWR* 48, no. 26 (9 July): 560–63.

Duclos, P., and B. J. Ward. 1998. Measles vaccines: A review of adverse events. *Drug Safety* 19, no. 6: 435–54.

Taylor B., E. Miller, C. P. Farrington, et al. 1999. Autism and measles, mumps and rubella vaccine: No epidemiological evidence for a causal association. *Lancet* 353, no. 9169 (12 June): 2026–29.

## Chapter 13: Chickenpox Vaccine

ACIP. 1996. Prevention of varicella: Recommendations of the ACIP. *MMWR* 45, no. RR-11 (12 July): 1–36.

———. 1999. Prevention of varicella: Update of Recommendations of the ACIP. *MMWR* 48, no. RR-6 (28 May).

CDC. 1999. Varicella-related deaths: Florida 1998. *MMWR* 48, no. 18 (14 May): 379–81.

## Chapter 14: Hepatitis A Vaccine

ACIP. 1999. Prevention of hepatitis A through active or passive immunization: Recommendations of the ACIP. *MMWR* 48, no. RR-12 (1 October).

## Chapter 16: Flu Vaccine

ACIP. 1999. Prevention and control of influenza: Recommendations of the ACIP. *MMWR* 48, no. RR-4 (30 April): 11.

Lasky, T., G. Terracciano, L. Magder, et al. 1998. Guillain-Barré Syndrome and the 1992–93 and 1993–94 influenza vaccines. *New England Journal of Medicine* 339:1797–1802.

## Chapter 17: Meningococcal Vaccine

ACIP. 1997. Control and prevention of meningococcal disease and control and prevention of Serogroup C meningococcal disease: Evaluation and management of suspected outbreaks. Recommendations of the ACIP. *MMWR* 46, no. RR-5 (14 February): 1–21.

———. 1999. Meningococcal disease and college students: Recommendations of the ACIP. Draft distributed during the public meeting of the ACIP in Atlanta (October).

CDC. 1999. Meningococcal disease: New England, 1993–1998. *MMWR* 48, no. 29 (30 July): 629–33.

Rosenstein, N.E., B. A. Perkins, D. S. Stephens, et al. 1999. The changing epidemiology of meningococcal disease in the United States, 1992–1996. *Journal of Infectious Diseases* 180, no. 6 (December): 1894–1901.

Jackson, L.A., A. Schuchat, R. D. Gorsky, and J.D. Wenger. 1995. Should college students be vaccinated against meningococcal disease? A cost-benefit analysis. *American Journal of Public Health* 85: 843–45.

———, and J. D. Wenger. 1993. Laboratory-based surveillance for meningococcal disease in selected areas: United States, 1989–1991. *MMWR* 42: 21–30.

**Chapter 19: Vaccines for Special Circumstances**

ACIP. 1999. Human rabies prevention: United States, 1999. Recommendations of the ACIP. *MMWR* 48, no. RR-1 (8 January): 1–21.

CDC. 1996. The role of BCG vaccine in the prevention and control of tuberculosis in the United States: A joint statement by the Advisory Council for the Elimination of Tuberculosis and the ACIP. *MMWR* 45, no. RR-4 (26 April): 1–18.

———. 1999. *Immunization of Adults: Your Call to Action.* Atlanta: DHHS.

———. 1999. Progress toward the elimination of tuberculosis: United States, 1998. *MMWR* 48, no. 33 (27 August): 732–36.

**Chapter 22: Vaccines and Bioterrorism: Smallpox and Anthrax**

The July–August 1999 issue of the CDC's journal *Emerging Infectious Diseases* focuses on bioterrorism. See http://www.cdc.gov/eid.

Questions on anthrax vaccination of the military can be addressed to the U.S. Department of Defense. Call (703) 697-5737 or see http://www.defenselink.mil/other_info/protection.html#Anthrax.

John Grabenstein presented data on anthrax vaccine reports to VAERS from 1990 to 1999 at the October 1999 public ACIP meeting in Atlanta.